OSCEs for the
MRCS PART B

A Bailey and Love Revision Guide

Bailey & Love
REVISION GUIDES

OSCEs for the
MRCS PART B

A Bailey and Love Revision Guide

JONATHAN M FISHMAN
BM BCh (Oxon), MRCS (Eng), DOHNS (RCS Eng), BA (Hons),
MA (Cantab)
ENT Specialist Registrar, The John Radcliffe Hospital, Oxford

VIVIAN A ELWELL
MB BS, MRCS, BA (Hons), MA (Cantab)
*Neurosurgery Specialist Registrar, The National Hospital for Neurology &
Neurosurgery, Queen Square, London*

RAJAT CHOWDHURY
BM BCh (Oxon), MRCS, BSc (Hons), MSc (Lond), MA (Oxon)
*Radiology Specialist Registrar, Southampton General Hospital,
Southampton*

All are Managing Directors of Insider Medical Ltd

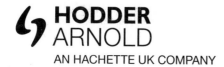
HODDER
ARNOLD
AN HACHETTE UK COMPANY

Hodder Arnold
A member of the Hodder Headline Group
First published in Great Britain in 2009 by
Hodder Arnold, an imprint of Hodder Education,
part of Hachette UK, 338 Euston Road, London NW1 3BH

http://www.hoddereducation.com

Whilst the advice and information in this book are believed to be true and accurate at the date of going to press, neither the author[s] nor the publisher can accept any legal responsibility or liability for any errors or omissions that may be made. In particular, (but without limiting the generality of the preceding disclaimer) every effort has been made to check drug dosages; however it is still possible that errors have been missed. Furthermore, dosage schedules are constantly being revised and new side-effects recognized. For these reasons the reader is strongly urged to consult the drug companies' printed instructions before administering any of the drugs recommended in this book.

British Library Cataloguing in Publication Data
A catalogue record for this book is available from the British Library

Library of Congress Cataloging-in-Publication Data
A catalog record for this book is available from the Library of Congress

ISBN   978-0-340-98580-9

2 3 4 5 6 7 8 9 10

Commissioning Editor:	Gavin Jamieson
Project Editor:	Sarah Penny
Production Controller:	Joanna Walker
Cover Design:	Helen Townson

Typeset in 10pt Formata Light Condensed by Phoenix Photosetting, Chatham, Kent
Printed and bound in India by Replika Press

What do you think about this book? Or any other Hodder Arnold title?
Please visit our website: www.hoddereducation.com

Contents

About the authors

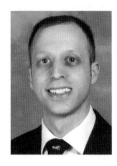

Jonathan M Fishman BM BCh (Oxon), MRCS (Eng), DOHNS (RCS Eng), BA (Hons), MA (Cantab)
Jonathan is an Oxford Specialist Registrar in ENT and a member of the Royal College of Surgeons. He graduated with a First Class Honours Degree in Natural Sciences from Sidney Sussex College, University of Cambridge, and completed his clinical training at St John's College, University of Oxford. He has held posts in Accident and Emergency, ENT, General Surgery and Neurosurgery, as part of the surgical rotation at St Mary's Hospital, Imperial College, London.

Jonathan has extensive teaching experience and is the primary author of three undergraduate and two postgraduate medical textbooks, including the highly successful *History Taking in Medicine and Surgery* (Pastest Publishing, 2005). He spent part of his medical training at both Harvard University and the NASA Space Center.

Jonathan was awarded Taylor and Howard-Agg Scholarships at Sidney Sussex College, Cambridge, and has been awarded the highly prestigious title of 'Lifelong Honorary Scholar' by the University of Cambridge, for academic excellence. He has been awarded a fellowship from the British Association of Plastic Surgeons for research at NASA, and from Cambridge University for research at Harvard University. Jonathan has recently been awarded the Royal Society of Medicine GlaxoSmithKline fellowship Award for his academic achievements to date and for demonstrating outstanding promise. He is committed to a career in academic ENT, with a strong emphasis on research and education.

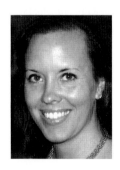

Vivian A Elwell MB BS, MRCS, BA (Hons), MA (Cantab)
Currently working as a Specialist Registrar in Neurosurgery, Vivian has held posts in Accident and Emergency, Orthopaedics, Neurosurgery and General Surgery with the surgical rotation at St Mary's Hospital, Imperial College, London.

She is an author of a best-selling undergraduate textbook, *Essential OSCE Topics for Medical and Surgical Finals* (Radcliffe Publishing, 2008). She taught clinical skills to medical students and doctors, and was an anatomy demonstrator at the Imperial College School of Medicine, London. She also served on the Imperial College School of Medicine Curriculum Development Committee.

Vivian's awards include the Swinford Edward Silver Medal Prize for her OSCE Examination, the Columbia University Research Fellowship at Columbia College of Physicians and Surgeons in New York City, the Columbia University King's Crown Gold and Silver Medal Awards, the Kathrine Dulin Folger Cancer Research Fellowship and the 'Who's Who of Young Scientists Prize'.

She earned a Bachelor's degree in biological sciences at Columbia

College, Columbia University, and an MA from the University of Cambridge. She gained Bachelor of Medicine and Bachelor of Surgery degrees from the Imperial College School of Medicine, and is a member of the Royal College of Surgeons.

Rajat Chowdhury BM BCh (Oxon), MRCS, BSc (Hons), MSc (Lond), MA (Oxon)

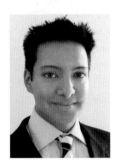

Rajat is a Specialist Registrar in Radiology and is a member of the Royal College of Surgeons. He was awarded an Honours degree in biological science from University College London, and completed his medical studies at Oxford University, the Mayo Clinic and Harvard University. He then trained on the surgical rotation at St Mary's Hospital, Imperial College, London, and held posts in Accident and Emergency, Orthopaedics and Trauma, Cardiothoracic Surgery, General Surgery, and Plastic Surgery.

Rajat has a diverse teaching record. He has taught clinical medicine to students and doctors in Oxford and London, and has tutored biochemistry and genetics to undergraduate students at Oxford University. He was an anatomy demonstrator at the Imperial College School of Medicine, London, and was President of the Queen's College Medical Society, Oxford, and of the Hugh Cairns Surgical Society.

Rajat's academic awards include Oxford University's Bristol Myers Squibb Prize in Cardiology, the Radcliffe Infirmary Prize for Surgery, the GlaxoSmithKline Medical Fellowship, the Warren Scholarship for Paediatric Studies at the University of Toronto, and the Exhibition Award to Harvard University. He is committed to a career in interventional and academic radiology. He has successfully completed Part 1 of the FRCR examinations, and is the lead author of the forthcoming undergraduate textbook, *Radiology at a Glance* (Wiley-Blackwell Publishing).

Acknowledgements

This book would not have been possible without the help of the following individuals:

Dr David S Fishman, Mrs Wendy F Fishman, Mrs Carole D Elwell, Mr and Mrs A Chowdhury, Miss M Chowdhury

Preface

This book has been written as an accompaniment to *Bailey and Love's Short Practice of Surgery* with the MRCS examination in mind. It is dedicated to the MRCS Part B Objective Structured Clinical Examination (OSCE), which is the final part of the Intercollegiate MRCS examination. This new examination was introduced in the autumn of 2008 and replaces the MRCS Part 3 Viva and Clinical Examination. It was developed to reflect the changes in postgraduate surgical training in the UK and is approved by the Postgraduate Medical Education Training Board (PMETB). This exam is designed and set by the Royal Colleges of Surgeons to test the knowledge, skills and attributes acquired during core surgical training. Successful completion of the MRCS will then allow surgical trainees to progress to ST3 in their chosen subspecialty.

Achieving success in the MRCS OSCE requires a thorough basic understanding of clinical medicine, professional examination and technical skills, problem-solving and decision-making, as well as excellent bedside manner and people skills. It is not difficult to appear hesitant and unintelligent under exam duress, even for the most gifted among us. However, a precise, structured and systematic approach can easily transform the nervous candidate into one who appears confident, dynamic and multi-dimensional. A planned strategic approach thus ensures that candidates are equipped with the essential tools to face any challenge they may face.

The MRCS OSCE can be likened to a circuit training course, in that the stations are quick and candidates must immediately switch into their new task at the ring of a bell. It is inevitable that adrenaline is running high but, in our experience, it is those candidates who channel these emotions in a positive way who emerge with a positive MRCS OSCE result.

This book is based on our highly successful *Insider Medical MRCS Part B OSCE Course*, and the feedback obtained from candidates who have sat the exam. We have therefore written this book with the aim of targeting high-yield topics that are likely to be faced and offer methods to tackle the challenges that may be posed in the exam. We have drawn from our breadth of experience of teaching at both the undergraduate and postgraduate levels and have identified common pitfalls. We therefore also include top tips on getting through those tricky situations which can often be the fine line between success and failure.

We are confident that this book will assist any trainee surgeon to sail through the MRCS OSCE with ease and we hope to make the time taken to prepare for the exam that much more enjoyable and rewarding. Our desired outcome is to secure the future of surgical science and practice, by guiding trainee surgeons in their quest for mastering their art.

Jonathan M Fishman
Vivian A Elwell
Rajat Chowdhury

Introduction

The MRCS Part B OSCE: an insider's guide to success

Successful completion of the MRCS Part A of the Intercollegiate MRCS examination allows passage to the MRCS Part B OSCE, which is your final stop on the road to becoming a member of one of the Royal Colleges of Surgeons. Furthermore, it marks reaching the landmark to be eligible to enrol on a programme that will train you to be an expert in your chosen subspecialty. The MRCS OSCE is a truly dynamic exam that demands an equally dynamic response from you to acknowledge your prowess in surgical science and art, as well as your skill and integrity.

Structure of the MRCS Part B OSCE

The MRCS Part B OSCE can be likened to a 3½ hour 'circuit course' comprising 16 examined stations and 4 additional rest periods. The exam covers the generic surgical curriculum, but candidates can now pre-select two specialty areas to be examined on from head and neck, trunk and thorax, limbs (including spine), and neurosciences. Consequently 4 of the 16 examined stations will be dedicated to these two chosen specialties.

Key features of the exam

- There are 16 examined stations in total, with 9 minutes for each.
- There are 4 rest or preparation stations, with 9 minutes for each.
- There are 5 subject disciplines areas across the 16 examined stations:
  - anatomy and surgical pathology (3 stations)
  - applied surgical science and critical care (3 stations)
  - surgical skills and patient safety (2 stations)
  - clinical skills in history taking and physical examination (5 stations)
  - communication skills (3 stations).
- Four of the 16 examined stations are specific to two specialties pre-selected by the candidate. The first specialty will be examined in one station of each of the following – anatomy and surgical pathology; clinical skills history taking; clinical skills physical examination. The second specialty will be examined in one station only – clinical skills physical examination.
- Twelve of the 16 examined stations are 'manned' (one or two examiners).
- Four of the 16 examined stations are 'unmanned' (1 station in anatomy and surgical pathology, 1 station in communication skills, 2 stations in applied surgical science and critical care). These may be written questions requiring written answers.
- There are 6 domains assessed in total across the 16 examined stations, but only up to 4 of these domains will be assessed in each individual station:
  - clinical knowledge
  - clinical skill

- technical skill (manual dexterity, hand/eye coordination)
- communication
- decision-making, problem-solving, situational awareness and judgement
- organisation and planning.

■ Each station is marked out of a total of 16 points and the entire exam is marked out of a total of 256 points.
■ Each station is further awarded a global rating for competence marked as:
  - fail
  - borderline fail
  - borderline pass
  - pass.

A candidate must achieve at least a 'borderline pass' in all 16 examined stations, regardless of the points total out of 256 points, to be awarded an overall 'pass' in the OSCE.

The mask of a professional

It is clear from the structure of the MRCS Part B OSCE that the experience of completing the exam is like being the only doctor in the hospital and managing the entire surgical division! You are required to be managing a trauma call one minute, breaking bad news in clinic the next, suturing a wound seconds later, followed immediately by engaging in academic debate over anatomical prosections, and you've only just started! Furthermore, you're not just trying to maintain your nerve and sanity, you are trying to appear unflustered, confident, and on top-form every step of the way. This is indeed a very tall order, so one of the most crucial parts of your preparation for this exam is trying to develop a flawless mask of professionalism, composure and control that cannot be removed regardless of the changing challenges that are thrown at you. It is only through maintaining placid composure that you will create the space to have clarity in thought to put together a strategic plan of action and answer questions intelligibly.

Many candidates are guilty of the common pitfall of spending disproportionate time on acquiring 'clinical knowledge' and are often careless and lack confidence in their approach. However, equal points are awarded for skill, communication, decision-making, organisation and planning. In many ways the clinical skills (physical examination) stations can be classed in the same genre as the driving test where an exaggerated display of the 'mirror, signal, manoeuvre' protocol is displayed for the benefit of the examiner. In most stations fastidious attention to basic protocol rituals, such as handwashing and appropriate patient introductions, will not only win favour of the examiners but will also score easy points that could make all the difference between failing and passing comfortably.

Practice makes perfect

The best preparation for this exam is to work with your fellow candidates as a team. You should unashamedly practise and critique each other's performance on systematic physical examinations, practical procedures, *viva voce*-style questioning, as well as discussing and rehearsing communication skills vignettes. You must practise until the step of handwashing, for example, becomes almost an automatic involuntary action. Moving through the exercise of history taking and physical examinations should become swift, smooth and natural so that you can then optimise your efforts on eliciting the salient signs. It is only in this way that you will feel confident to generate an appropriate differential diagnosis for what may seem like a baffling case when under the pressures of extreme exam stress.

Examiners will generally not interrupt or prompt you during the examination of patients and so it is up to you to move through the OSCE station picking up all the points available. The best way to achieve this is therefore planning every second of your 9 minute routine and practising it to pure perfection. It is only through rigorous rehearsal that a theatrical stage show is perfected for public performance and unforeseen mishaps are managed professionally on opening night.

A day in the life of an ST3

An important concept that you should consider is the benchmark your examiners are assessing you against. The MRCS Part B OSCE is a window into the life of you as a potential ST3 to see how you perform and if you are up to the task. You should therefore unofficially rename your preparation for the exam as 'preparing to be an ST3'. You should approach the exam with your 'ST3 hat' on and demonstrate appropriate levels of confidence, gravitas, maturity, safe decision-making and management skills, in addition to your core surgical knowledge and skill. Successful candidates are those who possess flair and finesse, deliver safe logical workups, and in essence portray themselves as a contender to take on the role as a Consultant's deputy.

Style over substance

The power of the first impression you create cannot be overestimated. How you look speaks volumes through your non-verbal communication. Modern infection control practices have impacted on dress codes for all healthcare professionals, and this now reflects in the exam. Some golden nuggets for portrayal as a responsible, respectable, knowledgeable and safe surgeon include:

For women:

- business blouse (bare below the elbows)
- minimal jewellery and makeup
- long hair tied back

- comfortable shoes
- antiperspirant and perhaps subtle perfume.

For men:
- business shirt (bare below the elbows)
- no tie
- recent smart haircut
- no jewellery (except wedding band)
- clean shoes
- antiperspirant and perhaps subtle aftershave.

The dress rehearsal

Revision courses that simulate the exam are excellent to give you a dry run. They can be done at any time but are probably best done when you are nearing the end of your preparation to highlight areas of refinement that can help to further raise your game. You can learn from your own mock exam experience, viewing others in action, and the feedback from the tutors and your colleagues. This is a time to allow others to critique your performance and point out any bad habits that you may be oblivious to. If you attend the course wearing the attire you are likely to be wearing on the day of the actual exam, you will reveal whether your shoes and clothes are comfortable for the 3½ hour OSCE experience.

One night to go

Preparation, of course, begins long before the big day. However, on the night before you should ensure your equipment that you want to take is ready and in order. All equipment that is required for the OSCE will be provided at the exam. However, for familiarity, you might like to take with you the following pieces of equipment:

- stethoscope
- tape measure
- pen torch
- tongue depressor
- opaque tube (e.g. Smartie tube) for transillumination
- tourniquet (for varicose veins)
- hat pins (for neurological examination)
- a piece of card for the ulnar nerve examination.

Remember, you should test run putting the equipment you want to carry in your assigned pockets and ensure you are still comfortable to conduct the tasks required. Equipment that falls out of your pockets during a physical examination may tarnish your slick image.

Arrange your travel itinerary as soon as possible, and men should get a smart haircut in the week preceding the exam. On the evening before the big day, you should recheck your itinerary and prepare any paperwork (you will need to take valid photo ID that must be produced when registering at the exam centre). It is a good idea to prepare your clothes, shoes and bag (including an antiperspirant if you are prone to anxiety-related perspiration). It is probably not a good idea to experiment with a new restaurant or hit the town but instead set your alarm clock slightly earlier than you comfortably need and then get a good night's rest.

The last few hours

The first test on the big day is not hitting the 'snooze' button when the alarm rings. It is much better to take your time in getting ready than raising your stress levels by oversleeping and then rushing to make the train. Once you're up, it is worth checking the travel updates and then washing and dressing. You should definitely have a proper breakfast because you will need all your energy to be on peak form for the rest of the day. Before you leave, glance in the mirror and tell yourself – you are an ST3!

As a surgical trainee and indeed an ST3, you should conduct yourself professionally and be polite and courteous at all times. After all you are potentially on display to the examiners before you even arrive at the exam centre, since they may be travelling on the same plane, train or bus as you. Examiners have a habit of sniffing out exam candidates, especially those who have their face buried in this book on the way to the exam!

Top tips for the exam

- Pay particular attention to the briefing before the start of the exam and follow the instructions exactly. You do not want to get noticed by your inability to follow instructions and disorganisation.
- Do not carry your mobile phone during the exam. This is a disciplinary offence.
- You cannot be too polite and courteous to patients.
- Do not forget to enter your candidate number in unmanned written answer stations.
- You must use the handwash gel before and after every clinical skills station.
- You must listen to the examiner's instructions carefully and follow his or her instructions precisely. If you are at all unclear on what is required of you, do not be afraid to ask the examiner to repeat or rephrase the question.
- Aim to maintain eye contact with the examiners when speaking to them.
- Keep your answers simple and clear. Always speak slowly and articulate decisively.
- You will not be interrupted or prompted unless the examiner wants to redirect you. If the examiners are trying to redirect you, do not continue in your current path. You must take the hint and follow their instructions.

- You should execute your well-oiled routine and give an exhibitionary performance. You will not be required to give a running commentary but you may do so if you prefer.
- Summaries must be concise and only contain salient positive and negative findings, followed by a differential diagnosis.
- If you feel one station has not gone particularly well, you must erase it from your mind and stop any ruminations in their tracks. It is imperative that you proceed to your next station unflustered and unphased. As an ST3 you may be required to lead a team safely through situations of crisis by maintaining excellent performance – so the show must go on!

The bottom line

Your key for entry into the surgeons' club lies in your ability to think and perform like an ST3! All the very best of luck!

Anatomy

Introduction

Many students find preparing for the anatomy part of the examination a daunting task. It has been many years since you were last in the dissection room and there seems to be a vast amount of material to learn in a short time. It is all too easy to spend all your revision time on anatomy alone, at the expense of other areas of the exam. Although the examiners place a lot of emphasis on anatomy (and rightly so, because you cannot be a surgeon without knowing your anatomy well), do not neglect other areas. Remember, you must pass all the other areas of the OSCE too in order to obtain an overall pass.

Here are a few top tips:
- Be concise and accurate in your answers.
- Do not comment on anything you have not been asked about.
- Be systematic and logical.
- Try to apply your answer to surgical practice. The emphasis now is on *applied* anatomy.
- Do not dig yourself into any holes!
- Images that you are asked to comment on in the exam may represent normal anatomy, so the emphasis is on pointing out the key anatomical features, rather than pathology! So, if you are asked to comment on a barium enema do not necessarily go looking for a stricture!

We would recommend that your preparations should include the following:
- Visit the dissection room prior to the exam and look at some prosections.
- Invest in a good atlas of anatomy.
- Know and be able to demonstrate surface anatomy.
- Familiarise yourself with the main bones (osteology).
- Be prepared to be handed 'props' in the exam – bones, prosections, images etc.
- Know well your 'specialty specific' area and the 'college favourites'.

Embryology

→ ## Changes at birth

What changes occur at birth?
Several important changes take place at birth.
- The urachus (allantois) becomes the single, median umbilical ligament.
- The umbilical arteries become the right and left, medial umbilical ligaments, respectively.

- The left umbilical vein becomes the ligamentum teres (round ligament) in the free edge of the falciform ligament.
- The ductus venosus becomes the ligamentum venosum.
- The ductus arteriosus becomes the ligamentum arteriosum.
- In 2 per cent of cases the vitello-intestinal duct may persist as a Meckel's diverticulum.
- The foramen ovale in most cases obliterates at birth to become the fossa ovalis, but remains patent into adulthood in some 20 per cent of cases.

Why is it important to know about changes at birth?

Aberrations of the normal developmental process may lead to pathology.

- Failure of the urachus (which normally connects the bladder to the umbilicus) to obliterate may lead to a urachal fistula, sinus, diverticulum or cyst, often with leakage of urine from the umbilicus.
- Failure of the ductus arteriosus to obliterate at birth leads to a patent ductus arteriosus, resulting in non-cyanotic congenital heart disease.
- In 2 per cent of cases, the vitello-intestinal duct persists as a Meckel's diverticulum, with its associated complications.
- In some 20 per cent of cases the foramen ovale fails to obliterate completely at birth, resulting in a patent foramen ovale. This may become the site for paradoxical embolism (where venous thrombus migrates and enters the systemic circulation through a patent foramen ovale), resulting in stroke.

→ ## Branchial arches

What are the branchial (pharyngeal) arches, clefts and pouches?

The branchial or pharyngeal arches are the mammalian equivalent of the gill arches in fish. In humans, there are five pairs of branchial arches that develop in a cranio-caudal sequence (equivalent to gill arches 1, 2, 3, 4, 6). The 5th branchial arch never forms in humans, or forms as a short-lived rudiment and promptly regresses.

Each arch contains a central cartilaginous element, striated muscle, cranial nerve and aortic arch artery, surrounded by ectoderm on the outside and lined by endoderm. The arches are separated externally by ectodermally lined branchial clefts and internally by endodermally lined branchial pouches.

- The 1st arch gives rise to the muscles of mastication.
- The 2nd arch gives rise to the muscles of facial expression.
- The 3rd and 4th arches give rise to the muscles of vocalisation and deglutition.
- The 6th arch gives rise to the intrinsic muscles of the larynx.

What are the clinical implications?

Certain key features concerning the branchial arches are worth remembering because of their clinical significance.

- The superior parathyroid glands develop from the 4th branchial pouch; the inferior parathyroids, along with the thymus, are 3rd pouch derivatives. Consequently, the inferior parathyroids may migrate with the thymus down into the mediastinum; hence its liability to end up in unusual positions.
- The tongue is derived from several sources. The anterior two-thirds of the tongue mucosa is a 1st arch derivative, whereas the posterior one-third is derived from the 3rd and 4th arches. The tongue musculature, in contrast, arises from occipital somite mesoderm. For this reason, the motor and sensory nerve fibres of the tongue are carried by separate sets of cranial nerves.
- The thyroid gland arises from between the 1st and 2nd arches as a diverticulum (thyroglossal duct) which grows downwards leaving the foramen caecum at its origin. Incomplete thyroid descent may give rise to a lingual thyroid, a thyroglossal duct cyst or a pyramidal thyroid lobe.
- Apart from the 1st branchial cleft (which forms the external ear), the other clefts are normally obliterated by overgrowth of the 2nd pharyngeal arch, enclosing the remaining clefts in a transient, ectoderm-lined, lateral cervical sinus. This space normally disappears rapidly and completely. It may persist in adulthood as a branchial cyst or fistula.

Name the muscles of mastication and describe their innervation.

There are four muscles of mastication:

- temporalis
- masseter
- medial pterygoid
- lateral pterygoid.

They are all 1st branchial arch derivatives and are therefore all innervated by the same nerve (mandibular division of trigeminal, or Vc).

Note that the buccinator muscle is regarded as a muscle of facial expression and is therefore a 2nd branchial arch derivative innervated by the facial (7th) cranial nerve. This is one of many situations in which a good knowledge of embryology – and especially the branchial arches – may help to predict the anatomy.

→ ## Gonadal development

Outline the development of the gonads.

During embryonic and fetal life, the testes and the ovaries both descend from their original positions at the 10th thoracic level. This explains the long course taken by the gonadal arteries and the site of referred pain from the gonads to the umbilicus (T10 dermatome).

Descent is genetically, hormonally and anatomically regulated and depends on a ligamentous cord known as the gubernaculum. Furthermore, descent of the testis through the inguinal canal into the scrotum depends on an evagination of peritoneum known as the processus vaginalis. This normally obliterates at birth.

How may descent go wrong?
Gonadal descent is a complicated process and there are many ways in which it can go wrong. Most commonly, an undescended – or maldescended – testis may occur (cryptorchidism). A patent processus vaginalis may lead to the formation of a congenital hydrocele, or inguinal hernia.

→ Meckel's diverticulum

What is a Meckel's diverticulum?
A Meckel's diverticulum is the anatomical remnant of the vitello-intestinal duct. In the developing fetus the vitello-intestinal duct connects the primitive midgut to the yolk sac and also plays a part in intestinal rotation.

The vitello-intestinal duct normally regresses between the fifth and eighth weeks of development, but in 2 per cent of individuals it persists as a remnant of variable length and location – known as a Meckel's diverticulum, named after Johann Friedrich Meckel who first described the embryological basis of this anomaly in the nineteenth century.

Most often it is observed as a 5 cm (2 inch) intestinal diverticulum projecting from the anti-mesenteric wall of the ileum, about 2 feet (60 cm) from the ileocaecal valve. It is about twice as common in males than in females. However, this useful mnemonic ('the rule of 2s') holds true only in two-thirds of cases; the length of the diverticulum is variable and its site may be more proximal.

What complications might a Meckel's diverticulum undergo?
It is estimated that 15–30 per cent of individuals with a Meckel's diverticulum develop symptoms from one of the following:

- intestinal obstruction
- gastrointestinal bleeding
- acute inflammation (Meckel's diverticulitis)
- perforation
- intussusception.

Its blind end may contain ectopic tissue, namely gastric mucosa (in 10 per cent of cases), liver, pancreatic tissue, carcinoid or lymphoid tissue. This is important because gastric mucosa contains parietal cells that secrete hydrochloric acid. Therefore ulcers can form within the diverticulum (like a peptic ulcer), causing bleeding.

Bowel obstruction may be caused by the trapping of part of the small bowel by a fibrous band (that represents a remnant of the vitelline vessels) connecting the diverticulum to the umbilicus. Symptoms may closely mimic appendicitis. Therefore if a normal-looking appendix is found at laparoscopy, or during an open appendicectomy, it is important to exclude a Meckel's diverticulum as a cause of the patient's symptoms. Mortality in untreated cases is estimated to be 2.5–15 per cent.

Exceptionally a Meckel's diverticulum may be found in an inguinal or a femoral hernia sac (Littre's hernia).

Head, neck and vertebral column

→ ## Thyroid gland

What is the blood supply to the thyroid gland?

The blood supply is by way of the superior thyroid artery (a branch of the external thyroid artery), the inferior thyroid artery (a branch of the thyrocervical trunk of the first part of the subclavian artery) and rarely the small thyroidea ima which arises from the aorta to supply the isthmus. Venous drainage is through the superior and middle thyroid veins to the internal jugular veins and via the inferior thyroid veins to the brachiocephalic veins (usually on the left). It is important to know about this when performing thyroid surgery.

Why does the thyroid gland move upwards with swallowing, and why is this clinically important?

The thyroid gland is an endocrine gland that sits at the base of the neck like a bow-tie. It consists of two lateral lobes and an isthmus which is attached via Berry's ligament to the 2nd to 4th tracheal rings. (It is not attached to the thyroid cartilage!)

The thyroid gland moves upwards with swallowing because:
- it is attached to the trachea by Berry's ligament
- it is invested within pretracheal fascia.

This is important clinically as it defines a swelling within the neck as being of thyroid origin.

What is the innervation to the muscles of vocalisation?

All the intrinsic muscles of the larynx are supplied by the recurrent laryngeal nerve of the vagus, with the exception of the important cricothyroid muscle, which is supplied by the external branch of the superior laryngeal nerve. Cricothyroid is the muscle which is principally concerned with altering voice pitch by altering the length of the vocal cords. Damage to the superior laryngeal or recurrent laryngeal nerves can occur during thyroid, parathyroid, oesophageal, carotid or aortic arch surgery, leading to changes in the character of the voice and even airway compromise (Semon's law).

How does the thyroid gland develop, and what is its clinical significance?

The embryology of the thyroid gland is clinically extremely important. It descends from the foramen caecum between the anterior two-thirds and posterior one-third of the tongue via the thyroglossal duct. Before reaching its final position in the neck it loops under the hyoid bone (Fig. 1.1).

Figure 1.1 ● (a) Descent of the thyroid gland to its usual position in the neck. (b) Thyroid development.

(a)

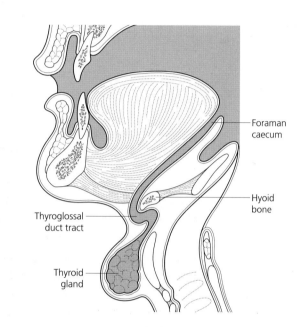

Foraman caecum

Hyoid bone

Thyroglossal duct tract

Thyroid gland

(b)

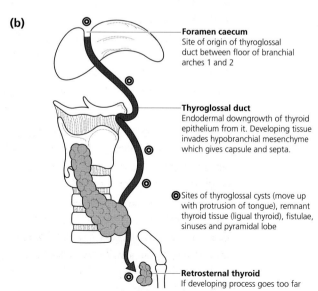

Foramen caecum
Site of origin of thyroglossal duct between floor of branchial arches 1 and 2

Thyroglossal duct
Endodermal downgrowth of thyroid epithelium from it. Developing tissue invades hypobranchial mesenchyme which gives capsule and septa.

◎ Sites of thyroglossal cysts (move up with protrusion of tongue), remnant thyroid tissue (ligual thyroid), fistulae, sinuses and pyramidal lobe

Retrosternal thyroid
If developing process goes too far

Note: The ultimobranchial bodies (5th pouch) give 'c' cells

An incompletely descended thyroid gland may persist into adult life as a lingual thyroid, a pyramidal thyroid lobe or a thyroglossal duct cyst. If it descends too far it can become a retrosternal thyroid. Thyroglossal duct cysts can become infected and form sinuses or fistulae.

In removing a thyroglossal duct it is important to remove the middle third of the hyoid bone and follow the tract up to the base of the tongue to prevent recurrence (Sistrunk's operation).

What does the thyroid gland do?

The thyroid gland is stimulated by the hormone TSH (which is produced from the anterior lobe of the pituitary gland) to produce T3 and T4. These are hormones that play an important role in basal metabolic rate.

→ Tongue

What is the innervation of the tongue (sensory and motor)?

Special taste sensation is by way of the chorda tympani division of the facial nerve for the anterior two-thirds of the tongue and the glossopharyngeal nerve for the posterior one-third. Taste on the anterior two-thirds of the tongue is therefore commonly lost in a facial nerve (or Bell's) palsy.

Somatic sensation is by way of the mandibular division of the trigeminal nerve for the anterior two-thirds of the tongue (lingual nerve) and the glossopharyngeal nerve for the posterior two-thirds.

All the muscles of the tongue are supplied by the hypoglossal (12th cranial) nerve, with the exception of the palatoglossus muscle which is supplied by the pharyngeal plexus of nerves (IX, X and sympathetics).

Name the muscles of the tongue.

Intrinsic muscles (wholly within the tongue and not attached to bone) are:

- longitudinal
- transverse
- vertical.

Extrinsic muscles (having a bony attachment) are:

- genioglossus
- styloglossus
- hyoglossus
- palatoglossus.

What type of epithelium is the tongue lined by?

The tongue is lined by stratified squamous (protective) epithelium as, like the skin, it is subject to 'wear and tear'. Tumours arising from the tongue are therefore typically squamous cell carcinomas.

→ Parathyroid glands

What are the parathyroid glands?

The parathyroid glands are pinkish brown glands usually found on the posterior aspect of the thyroid gland. In 90 per cent of individuals there are four, two on each side, but this varies from two to six. Each weighs about 50 mg and measures $6 \times 3 \times 2$ mm.

How do parathyroid glands develop?

The superior parathyroid glands are 4th branchial pouch derivatives, whereas the inferior parathyroids arise from the 3rd branchial pouch. The thymus gland is also a 3rd branchial pouch derivative. Therefore, the inferior parathyroid glands may get dragged down with the thymus into the mediastinum, making the position of the inferior parathyroid glands highly variable. The superior glands are more constant in position.

What is the blood supply of the parathyroid glands?

These glands are all usually supplied by the inferior thyroid artery. A consequence is that the inferior thyroid artery should always be preserved during a total thyroidectomy to prevent ischaemia of the parathyroid glands, which would render the patient hypocalcaemic, necessitating lifelong calcium supplementation.

What is the function of the parathyroid glands?

The glands secrete parathyroid hormone from chief (or principal) cells. Parathyroid hormone plays an essential role in calcium homeostasis. Calcitonin, on the other hand, is secreted by the parafollicular cells of the thyroid gland.

What does a general surgeon need to know about the parathyroids?

The parathyroids can produce too much hormone (hyperparathyroidism) or too little (hypoparathyroidism). Hypoparathyroidism usually follows thyroid or parathyroid surgery. Hyperparathyroidism can be primary, secondary or tertiary.

- Primary hyperparathyroidism usually results from a parathyroid adenoma, a benign tumour of usually one (but sometimes more than one) parathyroid gland that leads to the overproduction of parathyroid hormone and hypercalcaemia. Treatment consists of neck exploration and parathyroidectomy. Care must be taken to avoid damaging the recurrent laryngeal nerves. Exposure of the thymus through a midline sternotomy may rarely be necessary given the liability of the inferior parathyroid glands to end up in unusual positions. Less commonly primary hyperparathyroidism results from hyperplasia of the parathyroid glands or a carcinoma. In the case of the former, always think about multiple endocrine neoplasia.

- Secondary hyperparathyroidism is usually seen in the setting of chronic renal failure, where the levels of parathyroid hormone rise in response to a low calcium (remember that the kidney activates vitamin D).
- Tertiary hyperparathyroidism is commonly seen in renal transplant patients and results when the parathyroid glands become autonomously functioning.

What imaging modalities can be helpful in localising parathyroid adenomas preoperatively?

Preoperative localisation nowadays enables minimal-access surgery to be carried out. Helpful scanning modalities are:

- ultrasound scan
- Sestamibi isotope scan.

→ ## Skull base

How can the skull base be divided up?

There are three fossas:

- anterior cranial fossa
- middle cranial fossa
- posterior cranial fossa.

Name the structures running through the optic canal.

- Optic nerve
- Dural sheath
- Ophthalmic artery
- Sympathetics.

What runs through the superior orbital fissure?

- Ophthalmic division of trigeminal (Va) – lacrimal, frontal and nasociliary* branches
- Oculomotor nerve (III)*
- Trochlear nerve (IV)
- Abducent nerve (VI)*
- Sympathetic fibres
- Ophthalmic veins
- Branches of middle meningeal and lacrimal arteries

(* through tendinous ring).

What runs through the foramen magnum?

- Medulla
- Meninges
- Vertebral arteries with its sympathetic plexus
- Spinal roots of the accessory nerve
- Anterior spinal artery (formed from both vertebral arteries)
- Posterior spinal arteries

- Apical ligament of dens
- Tectorial membrane.

What runs through the foramen ovale?

- Mandibular division of the trigeminal (Vc)
- Lesser petrosal nerve
- Accessory meningeal artery.

What is the innervation of the extraocular muscles?

The extraocular muscles are innervated by the 3rd (oculomotor), 4th (trochlear) and 6th (abducent) cranial nerves. The trochlear nerve supplies only one muscle, the superior oblique muscle. The abducent nerve also supplies only one muscle, the lateral rectus muscle. This may be remembered by 'SO4, LR6'. All the remaining muscles are supplied by the oculomotor nerve – that is the superior rectus, inferior rectus, inferior oblique and medial rectus are all supplied by the oculomotor (3rd) cranial nerve. Injury to any of these cranial nerves (3rd, 4th or 6th) may result in ophthalmoplegia and diplopia.

The levator palpebrae superioris elevates the eyelid and has a dual innervation from both the oculomotor nerve and sympathetic fibres. The latter innervate a small smooth muscle portion of the levator muscle known as Muller's muscle. The clinical significance of this dual innervation is that a 3rd cranial nerve (oculomotor) palsy, or sympathetic interruption (Horner's syndrome), may result in ptosis.

To distinguish the two it is essential to lift up the eyelid and inspect the pupil to see whether it is enlarged (mydriasis in an oculomotor nerve palsy) or constricted (miosis in a Horner's syndrome). In an oculomotor palsy the eye points downwards and outwards from the unopposed action of superior oblique and lateral rectus, supplied by the 4th and 6th cranial nerves. Horner's syndrome is associated with hemifacial anhidrosis, flushing symptoms and enophthalmos, in addition to ptosis and miosis.

→ Posterior triangle of the neck

What are the borders of the posterior triangle of the neck?

- Posterior border of sternocleidomastoid
- Anterior border of trapezius
- Middle one-third of clavicle
- Roof of skin, platysma, investing layer of deep cervical fascia, external jugular vein
- Floor of prevertebral fascia covering muscles, subclavian artery, trunks of brachial plexus and cervical plexus.

What are the contents of the posterior triangle?

- *Nerves*: spinal root accessory, branches of cervical plexus
- *Arteries*: superficial (transverse) cervical, suprascapular, occipital

- *Veins*: transverse cervical, suprascapular, external jugular
- *Muscle*: omohyoid with sling
- *Lymph nodes*: level 5.

What is the course of the spinal accessory nerve?
The spinal accessory nerve is a branch of the 11th cranial nerve. It has been given the name spinal accessory since it originates from the upper end of the spinal cord (spinal roots, C1–C5). It passes through the foramen magnum and 'hitches a ride' with the cranial accessory nerve originating from the nucleus ambiguus. It passes out of the skull again by way of the jugular foramen. Its function is to supply only two muscles in the neck – the sternocleidomastoid and trapezius muscles.

What is the surface marking of the spinal accessory nerve?
The surface marking of the spinal accessory nerve is important. It traverses the posterior triangle of the neck from one-third of the way down the posterior border of the sternocleidomastoid muscle to one-third of the way up the anterior border of trapezius where it terminates (the 'rule of thirds'). It is vulnerable to iatrogenic injury in procedures that necessitate dissection within the posterior triangle of the neck, such as excision biopsy of a lymph node. In a radical en-bloc lymph node dissection of the neck for malignant disease, the spinal accessory nerve may have to be deliberately sacrificed in order to obtain satisfactory clearance.

What are the consequences of injury to the spinal accessory nerve in the posterior triangle of the neck?
Damage to this nerve leads to a predictive weakness of the trapezius muscle. This results in an inability to shrug the shoulder on the side in which the spinal accessory nerve is affected and may result in scapula winging. The sternocleidomastoid muscle is typically spared as the branch to the sternocleidomastoid is given off prior to the spinal accessory nerve entering the posterior triangle of the neck. The trapezius muscle also plays a role in hyperabduction of the arm and so activities such as combing one's hair would become more difficult. In the long term a trapezius palsy (with dropping of the shoulder) may result in a chronic, disabling neuralgia. This may occur as a result of pain from neurological denervation, adhesive capsulitis of the shoulder joint, traction radiculitis of the brachial plexus, or more commonly from fatigue.

→ ## Salivary glands

Name the salivary glands.
Major salivary glands are:
- parotid (predominantly serous exocrine secretion)
- submandibular (mixed mucinous and serous)
- sublingual (mainly mucinous exocrine secretion).

Minor salivary glands are scattered throughout the oral mucosa and submucosa (labial, buccal, palatoglossal, palatal and lingual).

What important structures lie within the parotid gland?

From superficial to the deep, these are important:

- five terminal branches of the facial nerve (also known as the pes anserinus, or 'goose's foot')
- retromandibular vein
- external carotid artery.

The facial nerve is the most superficial structure within the parotid gland and hence is extremely vulnerable to injury during parotid surgery. If the retromandibular vein comes into view, the facial nerve has already been severed! A facial nerve monitor should be used throughout and it is important to identify and protect the various branches of the facial nerve, which may be remembered by the mnemonic 'ten Zulus baited my cat' (from top to bottom):

- **t**en = **t**emporal branch
- **Z**ulus = **z**ygomatic branch
- **b**aited = **b**uccal branch
- **m**y = **m**arginal mandibular branch
- **c**at = **c**ervical branch.

The branches of the facial nerve are also likely to be injured by a malignant tumour of the parotid which is usually highly invasive and quickly involves the facial nerve, causing a facial paralysis.

Where does the parotid duct open?

The duct opens on the mucous membrane of the cheek opposite the 2nd upper molar tooth.

What is the secreto-motor innervation of the parotid?

The secreto-motor supply to the parotid (for secretion of saliva) is by way of parasympathetic fibres of the glossopharyngeal nerve (lesser petrosal nerve), synapsing in the otic ganglion and relaying onwards to the parotid gland through the auriculotemporal nerve.

What is Frey's syndrome?

A direct consequence of the innervation of the parotid gland is a phenomenon known as Frey's syndrome which may occur, not infrequently, following parotid surgery, or penetrating trauma to the parotid gland. It is caused by misdirected reinnervation of the auriculotemporal nerve fibres to the sweat glands in the facial skin following its injury. The patient may complain of gustatory sweating (i.e. sweating in response to a stimulus intended for saliva production).

What important nerves are at risk during a submandibular gland excision?

- Marginal mandibular division of the facial nerve

- Hypoglossal nerve
- Lingual nerve.

How can injury to the marginal mandibular nerve be avoided in a submandibular gland excision?

Injury to the marginal mandibular nerve can be avoided by:

- placing the incision two finger breaths beneath the angle of the mandible
- raising flaps deep to the investing layer of deep cervical fascia so that the nerve is safe by being pulled laterally in a superficial plane
- sectioning the facial vein low in the exposure and reflecting it superiorly, thereby drawing the marginal mandibular nerve superiorly away from the gland
- gentle traction to prevent stretching of the nerve
- intracaspular dissection of the gland
- minimising bleeding around the nerve and avoiding diathermy in close proximity to the nerve.

Use of a nerve stimulator facilitates identification of the marginal mandibular nerve through stimulation or contraction of the depressors to the ipsilateral lower lip.

→ Cavernous sinus

Summarise the walls of the cavernous sinus.

Note that the optic nerve is *not* contained within the cavernous sinus.

- *Roof*: anterior and posterior clinoid processes with uncus of temporal lobe and internal carotid artery on it, cranial nerves III and IV into it
- *Floor*: greater wing of sphenoid
- *Anterior wall* (narrow): medial end of superior orbital fissure, ophthalmic veins, orbit
- *Posterior wall* (narrow): dura of posterior fossa, superior and inferior petrosal sinuses, peduncle of brain
- *Medial wall*: dura over sphenoid, sella turica, pituitary, sphenoidal air sinus
- *Lateral wall*: dura, temporal lobe, cranial nerves III, IV, Va, Vb in wall (from top to bottom)
- *Contents*: internal carotid artery (with its associated sympathetic plexus), cranial nerve VI, blood.

What is meant by the 'danger area' of the face?

The area of facial skin bounded by the upper lip, nose, medial part of cheek and the eye is a potentially dangerous area to have an infection (the so-called 'danger area of the face'). An infection in this area may result in thrombosis of the facial vein, with spread of organisms through the inferior ophthalmic vein to the cavernous sinus. This may result in a cavernous sinus thrombosis. By the superficial middle cerebral vein, such thrombosis may spread to the cerebral hemisphere, which may be fatal unless adequately treated with antibiotics.

→ ## Circle of Willis

Draw the circle of Willis and label the different parts.
See Fig. 1.2.

Posteriorly:

- At the lower border of the pons, two vertebral arteries combine to form the basilar artery.
- At the upper border of the pons, the basilar artery terminates as right and left posterior cerebral arteries.

Anteriorly:

- Each internal carotid artery gives off an anterior and middle cerebral artery.
- The circle is completed anteriorly by the single, anterior communicating artery which connects the two anterior cerebral arteries.

The circle is completed posteriorly by the two posterior communicating arteries that connect the posterior cerebral arteries with the internal carotid arteries.

Where are most berry aneurysms situated?
See Fig. 1.2.

→ ## Fascial layers of the neck

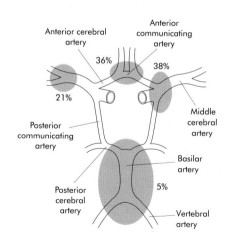

Figure 1.2 ● Main sites of intracranial supraclinoid aneurysms. (Bailey and Love, Figure 40.17a, p.635.)

What does the deep cervical fascia consist of?

- Investing layer of deep cervical fascia
- Pretracheal fascia
- Prevertebral fascia
- Carotid sheath.

What layers does one encounter when a tracheostomy is performed?

- Skin
- Subcutaneous fat
- Superficial fascia with platysma
- Investing layer of deep cervical fascia
- Strap muscles (sternohyoid muscle is encountered first, followed by sternothyroid)
- Pretracheal fascia
- Thyroid isthmus
- Trachea.

What does the carotid sheath contain?

- Internal jugular vein
- Carotid artery (common and internal parts)
- Vagus nerve
- Ansa cervicalis embedded within the anterior wall of the sheath overlying the internal jugular vein
- Lymph nodes.

Escaping from the upper part of the carotid sheath are the glossopharyngeal (IX), superior laryngeal branch of vagus (X), spinal accessory (XI) and hypoglossal (XII) nerves.

What are the branches of the external carotid artery?

- Superior thyroid
- Superficial temporal
- Maxillary
- Lingual
- Facial
- Ascending pharyngeal
- Posterior auricular
- Occipital.

Figure 1.3 ●
Branches of the
external carotid
artery

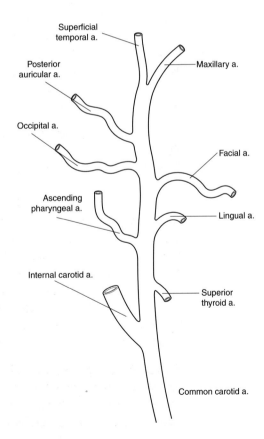

Superficial
temporal a.

Maxillary a.

Posterior
auricular a.

Occipital a.

Facial a.

Ascending
pharyngeal a.

Lingual a.

Internal carotid a.

Superior
thyroid a.

Common carotid a.

What structures lie at the C6 vertebral level?

- Cricoid cartilage
- Larynx – becomes trachea
- Pharynx – becomes oesophagus
- Vertebral artery – enters foramen transversarium of C6 vertebra
- Inferior thyroid artery and middle thyroid veins – cross to thyroid gland
- Middle cervical sympathetic ganglion
- Carotid tubercle of Chassaignac
- Omohyoid (superior belly) – crosses carotid sheath.

→ ## Spinal cord and vertebral column

What type of joint are the intervertebral joints?

They are secondary cartilaginous joints.

What type of joint is the sacro-iliac joint?

It is a synovial joint of the plane variety.

What does an intervertebral disc consist of?

Between each vertebral body lies an intervertebral disc which is made up of an annulus fibrosus of fibrocartilage, with an internal nucleus pulposus consisting of a semiliquid gelatinous substance derived from the embryonic notochord. With age the fibrocartilaginous annulus deteriorates and may weaken, often in the lower lumbar region, giving rise to a slipped, or prolapsed, disc. In such cases the nucleus pulposus is typically extruded posterolaterally.

What is the relationship of the nerve roots to the intervertebral discs?

The relationship of the nerve roots to intervertebral discs is of great importance. At the level of the L4/L5 disc, the 4th lumbar nerve roots within their dural sheath have already emerged from the intervertebral foramen and so are not lying low enough to come into contact with the disc. The roots that lie behind the posterolateral part of this disc are those of the 5th lumbar nerve and these are the ones likely to be irritated by the prolapse. Thus the general rule throughout the vertebral column is that when a disc herniates (usually posterolaterally, rather than in the midline) it may irritate the nerve roots numbered one below the disc. The exception to this rule is in cauda equina syndrome where the disc typically prolapses centrally rather then posterolaterally.

Where does the spinal cord end?

The spinal cord terminates at the level of L1/L2. Below this only nerve roots exist within the vertebral canal (cauda equina). It is therefore safe to perform a lumbar puncture at the level of L3/L4 or L4/L5. Fortunately for the purpose of a lumbar puncture, the dural sac containing the cerebrospinal fluid does not terminate until the level of S2.

What layers does one pass through when performing a lumbar puncture?

- Skin
- Superficial fascia
- Supraspinous ligament
- Interspinous ligament
- Ligamentum flavum
- Epidural space (loose areolar tissue containing internal vertebral venous plexus)
- Dura mater
- Arachnoid mater
- CSF in the subarachnoid space.

Thorax

→ Breast

Where does the breast lie anatomically?

The base of the breast is fairly constant; from the sternal edge to the midaxillary line and from the 2nd to the 6th ribs. Two-thirds of its base overlies pectoralis major and one-third overlaps onto serratus anterior. Contraction of the underlying pectoralis major muscle (by putting one's hands on the hips and pushing in) exacerbates any asymmetry between the breasts (e.g. as a result of a breast cancer) and is a clinically useful manoeuvre.

What is the blood supply to the breast?

Blood supply to the breast is mainly derived from the lateral thoracic artery (a branch of the second part of the axillary artery). However, the internal thoracic, thoraco-acromial and posterior intercostal arteries also send branches to the breast.

What is the breast's lymphatic drainage?

The lymphatic drainage of the breast is of considerable anatomical and surgical importance because of the frequent development of breast cancer and the subsequent dissemination of malignant cells along the lymphatics to the neighbouring lymph nodes. Around 75 per cent of the lymphatic drainage of the breast passes to roughly 20–30 axillary lymph nodes. They are usually described as lying in the following groups, which can be remembered by the mnemonic APICAL:

- A = anterior (or pectoral) group
- P = posterior (or subscapular) group
- I = infraclavicular (or deltopectoral) group
- C = central group

- **A** = apical group
- **L** = lateral (or brachial) group.

The medial quadrants of the breast (where fortunately cancer is less common) enter the thorax to drain into the internal mammary lymph nodes alongside the internal thoracic artery. Thoracic lymph nodes are difficult or impossible to treat, but lymph nodes of the axilla can be removed surgically.

The superficial lymphatics of the breast have connections with those of the opposite breast, anterior abdominal wall and supraclavicular lymph nodes. These tend to convey lymph from the breast when the other channels are obstructed by malignant disease, or following their destruction after radiotherapy or surgery.

→ Lungs

What are the contents of the lung hilum?
- Pulmonary artery
- Main bronchus
- Pulmonary vein
- Bronchial arteries and veins
- Lymph nodes and lymphatic channels
- Autonomics.

What is a bronchopulmonary segment?
There are typically 10 anatomically definable bronchopulmonary segments within each lung, each containing a segmental (tertiary) bronchus, a segmental artery, a segmental vein, lymphatics and autonomic nerves and separated from their adjacent segments by connective tissue. Each is pyramidal in shape with its apex towards the lung root and its base towards the surface of the lung, and each is anatomically and functionally separate from the rest. The surgical importance of this is that diseased segments, since they are structural units, can be selectively removed surgically (segmentectomy). Nowadays this can be performed by video-assisted thoracoscopic surgery (VATS).

How does the right main bronchus differ from the left?
The right bronchus is shorter, wider and more vertical than the left bronchus, so foreign bodies that fall down the trachea are more likely to enter the right bronchus. Furthermore, material aspirated by a supine, comatose or anaesthetised patient would tend to gravitate into the apical segment of the right lower lobe, which is consequently a common site for aspiration pneumonia and abscess formation.

What is the superior limit of the pleura?
The parietal pleura (along with the apex of the lung) projects 2.5 cm above the medial third of the clavicle superiorly. A penetrating wound above the medial end of the clavicle may therefore involve the apex of

the lung, resulting in a pneumothorax, or collapsed lung. This is most commonly seen as an iatrogenic complication during the insertion of a subclavian (central) venous line. Owing to the obliquity of the thoracic inlet, the pleura does not extend above the neck of the first rib, which lies well above the clavicle.

What is the lower limit of the pleura?

It is also important to remember that the lower limit of the pleural reflection, as seen from the back, lies below the medial border of the 12th rib, behind the upper border of the kidney. It is vulnerable to damage here during removal of the kidney (nephrectomy) through an incision in the loin. Proper identification of the 12th rib is essential to avoid entering the pleural cavity.

Demonstrate the surface anatomy of the pleural linings and lungs.

The reflections (and therefore the surface anatomy) of the pleural linings and lungs may be remembered by the '2, 4, 6, 8, 10, 12 rule'.

Pleura:

- Starts 2.5 cm above the midpoint of medial third of clavicle.
- Meet in midline at rib **2**.
- Left side diverges at rib **4** (to make room for the heart).
- Right side continues parasternally to rib **6**.
- Both cross rib **8** in midclavicular line.
- Both cross rib **10** in midaxillary line.
- Both reach posterior chest just below rib **12**.

Lungs:

Below rib 6, the lungs extend to two rib spaces less than pleura (i.e. opposite rib 6 in the midclavicular line, rib 8 in the midaxillary line, and rib 10 posteriorly). The parietal pleura extends a further two rib spaces inferiorly than the inferior lung edge to allow space for lung expansion.

Note how the right and left reflections are not identical to one another. On the left it is displaced by the central position of the heart.

→ Heart and pericardium

Outline the coronary artery circulation.

There are two principal coronary arteries – the right and the left. The right coronary artery originates from the anterior aortic sinus, whereas the left coronary artery originates from the left posterior aortic sinus. The left coronary artery divides into an anterior interventricular (or left anterior descending) artery and circumflex branches. The right coronary artery gives off the posterior interventricular (posterior descending) artery.

The right coronary artery supplies the right atrium and part of the left atrium, the sino-atrial node in 60 per cent of cases, the right ventricle, the posterior part of the interventricular septum and the atrio-ventricular node in 80 per cent of cases. The left coronary artery supplies the left atrium, left ventricle, anterior interventricular septum, sino-atrial node in 40 per cent of cases and the atrioventricular node in 20 per cent.

How many layers does the pericardium consist of?

There are three layers:

- outer fibrous pericardium
- inner serous pericardium (which comprises both an outer parietal layer and an inner visceral layer)

A small amount of pericardial fluid exists between the visceral and parietal layers of the serous pericardium. This allows the heart to move freely within the pericardial sac.

What are the pericardial sinuses?

Between the parietal and visceral layers there are two important pericardial sinuses. The transverse sinus lies in between the pulmonary artery and aorta in front and the pulmonary veins and superior vena cava behind. The oblique sinus is a space behind the heart between the left atrium in front and the fibrous pericardium behind, posterior to which lies the oesophagus.

The transverse sinus is especially important in cardiac surgery. A digit and ligature can be passed through the transverse sinus and, by tightening the ligature, the surgeon can stop the blood flow through the aorta or pulmonary trunk while cardiac surgery is performed.

→ Oesophagus

Describe the course of the oesophagus.

The oesophagus is a segmental muscular tube running from the cricoid ring, at the level of C6, to the cardia of the stomach. It is 25 cm long (with the distance from the upper incisor teeth to the lower oesophageal sphincter being approximately 40 cm). These distances are useful to learn for the purposes of endoscopy. The upper one-third of the oesophagus consists of skeletal muscle (voluntary muscle which initiates swallowing) but then there is a progressive change to smooth muscle, such that the lower third of the oesophagus consists only of smooth muscle.

What is the blood supply and lymphatic drainage of the oesophagus?

Blood supply and lymphatic drainage is segmental.

- The upper third of the oesophagus is supplied by the inferior thyroid artery and lymphatics drain to the deep cervical group of lymph nodes.
- The middle third of the oesophagus is supplied directly by branches from the descending thoracic aorta and lymphatics drain to the pre-aortic and para-aortic lymph nodes.

- The lower third of the oesophagus is supplied by the left gastric artery and lymphatics drain to the coeliac group of lymph nodes. However, within the oesophageal walls there are lymphatic channels which enable lymph to pass for long distances within the viscus, so that drainage from any given area does not strictly follow the above pattern.

What type of epithelium lines the oesophagus?

The surface epithelium is largely non-keratinising stratified squamous epithelium. This is normally replaced by columnar epithelium at the gastro-oesophageal junction, but columnar epithelium may line the lower oesophagus. An oesophagus that has the squamocolumnar junction 3 cm or more above the gastro-oesophageal junction is abnormal and called Barrett's oesophagus. This is a metaplastic change taking place in response to acid reflux and is a pre-malignant condition.

Identify the main sites of constrictions along the oesophagus.

- 15 cm from the incisor teeth, at the cricopharyngeus sphincter. The sphincter prevents air entering the oesophagus and stomach and relaxes with the swallowing reflex. This is the narrowest part of the oesophagus
- 22 cm from the incisor teeth, where the oesophagus is crossed by the aortic arch
- 27 cm from the incisor teeth, where the oesophagus is crossed by the left principal bronchus
- 38 cm from the incisor teeth, where the oesophagus passes through the opening in the diaphragm.

These measurements are important clinically with regard to the passage of instruments along the oesophagus. They are also sites where swallowed foreign bodies can lodge and where strictures commonly develop.

What factors contribute to the maintenance of the lower oesophageal sphincter?

The lower oesophageal sphincter is not a true anatomical sphincter, but rather a functional one. Maintenance of the lower oesophageal sphincter is largely brought about by the following:

- the effect of the right crus of the diaphragm forming a 'sling' around the lower oesophagus
- the oblique angle the oesophagus takes on entering the gastric cardia (Angle of His) acting as a 'flap valve' mechanism
- raised intra-abdominal pressure acting to compress the abdominal part of the oesophagus
- mucosal rosette (prominent folds at the gastro-oesophageal junction)
- phrenico-oesophageal ligament (a fold of connective tissue)
- the effect of gastrin in increasing lower oesophageal sphincter tone
- antegrade unidirectional peristalsis

- normal gastric motility and emptying
- swallowed saliva (lubrication and neutralisation).

A dysfunctional lower oesophageal sphincter may lead to problems, such as gastro-oesophageal reflux disease, hiatus hernia, or achalasia.

What is unique about the wall of the oesophagus?

Except for the short intra-abdominal segment of the oesophagus, there is no serosal surface, unlike the rest of the gastrointestinal tract (with the exception of the distal rectum). The consequences of this are two-fold. First, oesophageal anastomoses are particulary prone to leakage, because not only are the anastomoses technically difficult, but also the lack of a peritoneal covering to the oesophagus, with the rather friable oesophageal musculature, means the sutures rely for much of their tensile strength on the mucosa and submucosal layers. Second, because the oesophagus lacks a serosal covering, oesophageal carcinoma encounters few anatomic barriers to local invasion.

What are the characteristic manometric features of achalasia?

- Hypertensive lower oesophageal sphincter
- Non-relaxing lower oesophageal sphincter
- Aperistalsis.

→ ## Diaphragm

What is the diaphragm?

The diaphragm is a musculotendinous structure composed of outer skeletal muscle fibres and a central tendinous region. It partitions the thoracic from the abdominal cavity and is the main muscle of respiration at rest (accounting for 70 per cent of inspiration at rest).

What is the innervation of the diaphragm?

The diaphragm receives motor innervation from the phrenic nerve (C3, C4, C5). (C3, C4, C5 keeps the diaphragm alive!) The diaphragm has no other motor supply other than the phrenic nerve. This is why high cervical spine injuries can be so disastrous and hence the importance of proper cervical spine immobilisation in trauma victims.

The phrenic nerve is two-thirds motor and one-third sensory. The sensory nerve supply to the diaphragmatic parietal pleura and diaphragmatic peritoneum covering the central surfaces of the diaphragm is from the phrenic nerve. The sensory supply to the periphery of the diaphragm is from the lower six intercostal nerves.

What passes through the various openings in the diaphragm?

This is a common question! The answers are in Table 1.1.

Table 1.1
Openings through the diaphragm

Vena cava opening (T8)	Inferior vena cava Right phrenic nerve
Oesophageal opening (T10)	Oesophagus Left and right vagus nerves (RIP = **r**ight **i**s **p**osterior) Oesophageal branches of left gastric vessels Lymphatics from lower third of oesophagus
Aortic opening (T12)	Aorta Azygous and hemiazygous veins Thoracic duct
Crura (T12)	Greater, lesser and least splanchnic nerves
Behind medial arcuate ligament	Sympathetic trunks
Behind lateral arcuate ligament	Subcostal (T12) neurovascular bundle

N.B. The left phrenic nerve pierces the muscle of the left dome of the diaphragm.

Does the inferior vena cava pass through the muscular or tendinous portion of the diaphragm?

The inferior vena cava passes through the central tendinous portion of the diaphragm at the level of T8. If the vena cava passed through the muscular part of the diaphragm, every time the diaphragm contracts with respiration it would impede venous return causing syncope.

→ ## Thoracic duct

What is the course of the thoracic duct?

The thoracic duct is 45 cm long and commences at T12 from the cisterna chyli which lies to the right of the aorta.

■ It ascends behind the right crus and to the right of the aorta and oesophagus.
■ It crosses the midline to the left, posterior to the oesophagus, at the level of T5.
■ It passes over the dome of the left pleura, anterior to the left vertebral and subclavian arteries and enters the confluence of the left subclavian and internal jugular veins.

Valves are present along the duct and encourage the propagation of chyle along the duct.

What areas does the thoracic duct drain?

It drains all lymph below the diaphragm, left thorax, left head and neck regions.

What is the equivalent on the contralateral side?

The equivalent to the thoracic duct on the right is the right lymphatic trunk. This drains on the right into the confluence of the right subclavian and internal jugular veins.

Why do surgeons need to know about the thoracic duct?

Injury to the thoracic duct may occur following trauma, or during insertion of a central venous line. This may result in a chylothorax. The thoracic duct may also be injured in a neck dissection, resulting in a chyle leak.

Abdomen and pelvis

→ Transpyloric plane of Addision

What important structures traverse the transpyloric plane of Addison?

The transpyloric plane (of Addison) is an important landmark. It lies half way between the suprasternal notch and the symphysis pubis at the level of L1. It coincides with the following:

- L1 vertebra
- fundus of gallbladder
- hilum of kidneys
- hilum of spleen
- pylorus of the stomach (hence the name transpyloric)
- termination of the spinal cord in adults
- neck of pancreas
- origin of the portal vein
- origin of the superior mesenteric artery
- duodenojejunal flexure
- attachment of the transverse mesocolon
- tip of the 9th costal cartilage.

→ Peritoneal cavity

Where is the epiploic foramen of Winslow, and what are its boundaries?

This is the site at which the greater and lesser sacs of the peritoneal cavity communicate with one other. Its boundaries can be described as follows:

- *Anteriorly*: the lesser omentum with the common bile duct, portal vein and common hepatic artery in its free edge
- *Posteriorly*: inferior vena cava
- *Superiorly*: the caudate lobe of the liver
- *Inferiorly*: first part of the duodenum
- *Medially*: lesser sac (posterior to stomach)
- *Laterally*: greater sac.

What is the clinical significance of the epiploic foramen of Winslow?

■ It may be the site of internal herniation of bowel.
■ Compression of the common hepatic artery in the free edge of the lesser omentum by a carefully placed hand in the epiploic foramen may be a life-saving manoeuvre at laparotomy to control bleeding from the liver (Pringle's manoeuvre).

What three features distinguish large bowel from small bowel?

The following three features distinguish large bowel from small bowel in the cadaver, at laparotomy and on imaging. Large bowel has:

■ haustra (also known as sacculations)
■ appendices epiploicae
■ taenia coli.

Valvulae conniventes (synonymous with plicae circulares) are a feature of small bowel rather than large bowel.

What spaces are there within the peritoneal cavity?

The most important spaces to recognise are:

■ right and left subphrenic (subdiaphragmatic) spaces
■ right subhepatic space (also known as the hepatorenal pouch of Rutherford-Morison)
■ right and left paracolic gutters
■ pelvis.

These are potential sites for an intra-abdominal collection. When lying supine, the hepatorenal pouch is the most dependent part of the peritoneal cavity and hence is an area where intraperitoneal fluid is likely to accumulate in the form of an abscess (or 'collection'). The left subhepatic space is the lesser sac.

How many layers does the greater omentum consist of?

The greater omentum (or gastrocolic omentum) is a double sheet of peritoneum, fused and folded on itself to form an integral structure comprising four layers. The anterior two layers descend from the greater curvature of the stomach where they are continuous with the peritoneum on the anterior and posterior surfaces of the stomach. Posteriorly, they ascend up to the transverse colon where they loosely blend with the peritoneum on the anterior and posterior surfaces of the transverse colon and the transverse mesocolon above it.

What is the blood supply of the greater omentum?

The right and left gastro-epiploic arteries run between the layers of the greater omentum and supply it, close to the greater curvature of the stomach.

How may the lesser sac be approached?

There are various approaches:

Figure 1.4 ●
Arterial blood
supply of the
stomach.

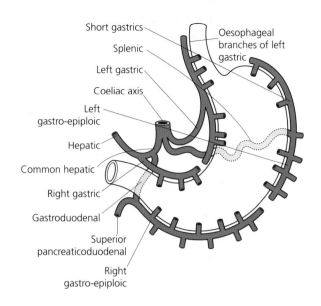

■ through the greater omentum (by incising between the greater
curvature of the stomach and the transverse colon and lifting the
stomach up)
■ through the lesser omentum
■ through the transverse mesocolon
■ through the epiploic foramen of Winslow
■ through either the gastrosplenic or lienorenal ligaments.

→ Blood supply of the stomach

Draw the blood supply to the stomach.
See Fig. 1.4.
The blood supply to the stomach may be easily remembered by a few
simple rules:

Rule 1
The coeliac trunk divides into three main branches, which can be easily
remembered by the mnemonic LHS ('left hand side'):
■ left gastric artery (L)
■ common hepatic artery (H)
■ splenic artery (S).

Rule 2
Divide the stomach up into three main areas:
■ lesser curvature

■ greater curvature
■ fundus.

Rule 3

The lesser curvature is supplied by the left and right gastric arteries. The left gastric as already mentioned comes directly off the celiac trunk. The right gastric is a branch of the common hepatic artery.

Rule 4

The greater curvature is supplied by the right and left gastro-epiploic arteries. The right gastro-epiploic artery comes off the gastroduodenal artery. The left gastro-epiploic artery comes off the splenic artery.

Rule 5

The fundus is supplied by the six (or so) short gastric arteries which arise from the splenic artery.

Rule 6

The gastroduodenal artery is an important artery. It arises from the common hepatic artery and lies posterior to the first part of the duodenum. A posteriorly placed duodenal ulcer may erode through the duodenal wall into the blood vessel, causing catastrophic, life-threatening haemorrhage. Urgent endoscopy or laparotomy may be required to stop the bleeding.

→ Gallbladder

What is the surface landmark of the gallbladder?

It is opposite the tip of the right 9th costal cartilage, that is, where the lateral edge of the right rectus sheath crosses the costal margin. This is an important landmark as it is the site of maximal abdominal tenderness in gallbladder disease.

What is the function of the gallbladder?

The gallbladder has three main functions – it stores bile, concentrates bile (5–20-fold), and adds mucous to the bile secreted by the liver. It has a capacity of about 50 mL. Its mucous membrane is a lax areolar tissue lined with simple columnar epithelium. Under the epithelium there is a layer of connective tissue, followed by a muscular wall that contracts in response to cholecystokinin, a peptide hormone secreted by the duodenal mucosa in response to the entry of fatty foods into the duodenum.

What is Calot's triangle?

It is the triangle formed by the liver edge, common hepatic duct and cystic duct. Calot's triangle reliably contains the cystic artery, the cystic lymph node (of Lund), connective tissue and lymphatics. It is important to dissect out this triangle at laparoscopic cholecystectomy in order to successfully identify and ligate the cystic artery prior to removal of the gallbladder.

How does gallstone disease refer pain to the shoulder?

Gallstone disease may refer pain to the right shoulder tip (Kehr's sign). There is an important anatomical explanation underlying this phenomenon. An inflamed or distended gallbladder may irritate the diaphragm which is supplied by the phrenic nerve (C3, C4, C5 keeps the diaphragm alive!). These very same nerve roots also provide sensation to the right shoulder tip by way of the supraclavicular nerves (C3–C5). The body misinterprets the signals that it receives and interprets the pain signals as coming from the right shoulder tip.

What is Courvoisier's law?

Courvoisier's law states that, in the presence of obstructive jaundice, a palpable gallbladder is unlikely to be due to gallstones. The reason is that gallstones cause chronic inflammation, fibrosis and a shrunken gallbladder. Note, however, that the law does not hold true in reverse (i.e. in the presence of obstructive jaundice, an impalpable gallbladder is always due to gallstones) as 50 per cent of dilated gallbladders cannot be palpated on clinical examination, due to patient obesity or because of overlap of the liver.

What factors favour the formation of cholesterol gallstones?

- Bile stasis
- Supersaturation of bile with cholesterol (lithogenic bile)
- Nucleation factors.

→ Portosystemic anastomoses

What are the sites of portosystemic anastomoses?

Portosystemic anastomoses are sites at which the portal venous circulation meets the systemic venous circulation. There are five principal sites where this takes place:

- lower oesophagus
- upper anal canal
- periumbilical region of the anterior abdominal wall
- bare area of the liver
- retroperitoneum.

What is the significance of the portosystemic anastomosis at the lower end of the oesophagus?

The veins from the lower third of the oesophagus drain downwards to the left gastric vein (portal system) and above this level oesophageal veins drain into the azygous and hemiazygous systems (systemic system). Subsequently in portal hypertension dilatations of the veins within the lower end of the oesophagus may take place, resulting in oesophageal varices. These can cause life-threatening haemorrhage.

What is the significance of the portosystemic anastomosis within the anterior abdominal wall?

Dilatations of veins within the anterior abdominal wall may result. These are known as caput medusae, because of their resemblance to the hair of the Greek mythological character, Medusa.

What is the significance of the portosystemic anastomosis within the anal canal?

Venous dilatations within the upper end of the anal canal in portal hypertension may lead to the formation of haemorrhoids. However, in practice, they rarely lead to problems and the presence of oesophageal varices is far more significant.

→ ## Spleen

What are the anatomical features of the spleen?

The spleen, the largest of the lymphoid organs, lies under the diaphragm on the left side of the abdomen. It may be summarised by '1, 3, 5, 7, 9, 11'. That is, it measures $1 \times 3 \times 5$ inches ($2.5 \times 7.5 \times 12.5$ cm), weighs 7 ounzes (200 g) and lies beneath the 9th to 11th ribs. The spleen lies at the far left extremity of the lesser sac beneath the diaphragm.

It is essential to understand the anatomical relations of the spleen (e.g. the pancreatic tail, stomach, splenic flexure of the colon, left kidney, diaphragm) in order to prevent inadvertent injury to these at splenectomy.

What are splenunculi?

Accessory spleen (splenunculi) represent congenital ectopic splenic tissue and are found in up to 20 per cent of individuals. One or several may be found, usually along the splenic vessels or in the peritoneal attachments. They are rarely larger than 2 cm in diameter.

What are the functions of the spleen?

The functions of the spleen may be summarised by FISH:

- **F** = **f**iltration and removal of old blood cells and encapsulated microorganisms
- **I** = **i**mmunological functions (production of IgM and opsonins)
- **S** = **s**torage function (30 per cent of the total platelets are situated within the spleen)
- **H** = **h**aematopoiesis (in the developing fetus).

It has recently been evoked that the spleen has an endocrine function through the production of an immuno-potentiating peptide called tuftsin.

What are the gastrosplenic and lienorenal ligaments?

Two 'pedicles', the gastrosplenic and lienorenal ligaments, connect the hilum of the spleen to the greater curvature of the stomach and the anterior surface of the left kidney, respectively. The splenic vessels and pancreatic tail lie in the lienorenal ligament. The short gastric and left gastro-epiploic vessels run in the gastrosplenic ligament.

What organisms are patients susceptible to after splenectomy?

Splenectomised patients are at high risk of postsplenectomy sepsis, especially from encapsulated organisms such as:

- *Haemophilus influenzae*
- *Neisseria meningitidis* (meningococcus)
- *Streptococcus pneumoniae* (pneumococcus).

They are prevented by administering the relevant vaccinations and giving prophylactic penicillin. Patients are also at risk of malaria (especially *Plasmodium falciparum*).

→ Adrenal glands

Describe the anatomical features of the adrenal glands.

The adrenal glands lie antero-superior to the upper part of each kidney. They weigh approximately 5 g each and measure 50 mm vertically, 30 mm across and 10 mm thick. They are somewhat asymmetrical, with the right adrenal being pyramidal in shape and left adrenal being crescentic, and lie within their own compartment of (Gerota's) renal fascia. A fascial septum separates the adrenal gland from the kidney – which explains why in nephrectomy (removal of the kidney) the latter gland is not usually displaced (or even seen).

What is the blood supply to the adrenal glands?

Each gland, although weighing only a few grams, has three arteries supplying it – a direct branch from the aorta, a branch from the renal artery and a branch from the inferior phrenic artery. This reflects the high metabolic demands of the tissue.

What is the venous drainage of the adrenals?

The single main suprarenal vein drains into the nearest available vessel – on the right it drains into the inferior vena cava and on the left directly into the renal vein. The right adrenal gland is tucked medially behind the inferior vena cava. In addition, the right suprarenal vein is particularly short and stubby. Both these features make the inferior vena cava vulnerable to damage in a right adrenalectomy.

What are the different layers of the adrenal gland and what do they produce?

The adrenal gland comprises an outer cortex and an inner medulla, which represent two developmentally and functionally independent endocrine glands within the same anatomical structure. The medulla is derived from the neural crest (ectoderm). It receives preganglionic sympathetic fibres from the greater splanchnic nerve and secretes adrenaline (70 per cent) and noradrenaline (30 per cent). The cortex is derived from mesoderm and consists of three layers, or zones. The layers from the surface inwards may be remembered by the mnemonic GFR:

- **G** = zona **g**lomerulosa (secretes aldosterone)
- **F** = zona **f**asciculata (secretes cortisol and sex steroids)
- **R** = zona **r**eticularis (secretes cortisol and sex steroids).

→ ## Appendix

What is the blood supply to the appendix?

The appendicular artery provides the supply, being a branch of the ileocolic artery which arises from the superior mesenteric artery.

What is the surface landmark of the appendix?

The surface marking of the base of the appendix is situated one-third of the way up the line joining the anterior superior iliac spine to the umbilicus (McBurney's point). This is an important landmark when making an appendicectomy (McBurney's or gridiron) incision.

Where may the appendix be found?

The position of the free end of the appendix is very variable. The most common, as found at operation, is the retrocaecal or retrocolic position (75 per cent of cases), with the subcaecal or pelvic position next in order of frequency (20 per cent of cases). Less commonly, in 5 per cent of cases, it lies in the pre-ileal or retro-ileal positions, or lies in front of the caecum, or in the right paracolic gutter.

What layers are encountered by the surgeon when performing an appendicectomy?

- Skin
- Subcutaneous tissue (Camper's fascia)
- Scarpa's fascia
- External oblique aponeurosis
- Internal oblique
- Transversus abdominis
- Transversalis fascia
- Preperitoneal (extraperitoneal) fat
- Parietal peritoneum.

Why does appendicitis commonly cause periumbilical pain?

Afferent nerve fibres concerned with the conduction of visceral pain from the appendix accompany the sympathetic nerves and enter the spinal cord at the level of T10. Consequently, the appendix refers visceral pain to the T10 dermatome which lies at the level of the umbilicus. Only later, when the parietal peritoneum overlying the appendix becomes inflamed, does the pain become more intense and localise to the right iliac fossa in the region of McBurney's point.

→ ## Rectum

Where does the rectum begin and end?

The rectum is 12 cm long, starting at the level of S3 and ending at the puborectalis (levator ani-pelvic floor).

Describe the peritoneal reflections of the rectum.

The rectum has no mesentery and is therefore regarded as retroperitoneal. It is covered by peritoneum on its front and sides in its upper third, only on its front in its middle third and the rectum lies below the peritoneal reflection in its lower third. Do not be confused; although the rectum has no mesentery, the visceral pelvic fascia around the rectum is often referred to by surgeons as the mesorectum. The pararectal lymph nodes are found within the mesorectum, which is removed together with the rectum as a package during rectal excision for carcinoma.

What is the blood supply of the rectum?

Blood supply is by way of the superior rectal (inferior mesenteric), middle rectal (internal iliac) and inferior rectal (internal pudendal) arteries. The venous drainage is as for the arteries. Note, however, that there is a portosystemic anastomosis in the lower rectal and upper anal canal walls, as branches of the superior rectal (portal) and inferior/middle rectal veins (systemic) meet in the external and internal venous plexuses. This may result in haemorrhoids in portal hypertension.

What is the nerve supply to the rectum?

The rectum receives parasympathetic nerve fibres from the pelvic splanchnic nerves, or nervi erigentes, originating from S2–S4. It functions to relax the internal sphincter, contract the bowel and transmit a sense of fullness. Note that the vagus nerve supplies bowel only up to two-thirds along the transverse colon. The whole of the rest of the bowel inferior to this level (the so-called hindgut) receives parasympathetic fibres by way of the pelvic splanchnic nerves.

Sympathetic supply to the rectum is through the lumbar splanchnics and superior hypogastric plexus. Sympathetics contract the internal sphincter, relax the bowel and transmit visceral pain.

→ Inguinal canal

What are the boundaries of the inguinal canal?

- *Anterior wall*: skin, superficial fascia, external oblique (for whole length); internal oblique for lateral one-third
- *Posterior wall*: transversalis fascia (for whole length); conjoint tendon and pectineal (Cooper's) ligament medially
- *Floor*: inguinal ligament (Poupart's ligament)
- *Roof*: arching fibres of internal oblique and transversus abdominis which fuse to form the conjoint tendon on the posteromedial aspect of the canal.

The deep inguinal ring is a hole in the transversalis fascia and lies a finger-breadth above the mid-inguinal point (i.e. half way between the anterior superior iliac spine and pubic tubercle). The superficial inguinal ring is a hole in the external oblique aponeurosis.

What is a hernia?
A hernia is a protrusion of a viscus, or part of a viscus, outwith its normal position.

How can you distinguish a femoral from an inguinal hernia?
An inguinal hernia lies above and medial to the pubic tubercle, while a femoral hernia lies below and lateral to the pubic tubercle.

What is the difference between a direct and an indirect inguinal hernia?
A direct hernia passes straight through a weakness in the anterior abdominal wall and passes through the superficial ring only. An indirect hernia passes through both the deep and superficial inguinal rings and thereby passes along the entire length of the inguinal canal. They can be distinguished clinically by placing your hand over the deep ring and asking the patient to cough (deep ring occlusion test). An indirect hernia is controlled at the deep ring, whereas a direct inguinal hernia is not.

At surgery, the neck of an indirect inguinal hernia lies lateral to the inferior epigastric artery, whereas the neck of a direct inguinal hernia lies medial to the inferior epigastric artery. Occasionally a pantaloon hernia may occur (with both direct and indirect components).

What is Hasselbach's triangle, and what is its surgical importance?
The boundaries of Hasselbach's triangle are:
- medial half of inguinal ligament
- linea semilunaris (lateral border of rectus abdominis)
- inferior epigastric artery.

Its surgical importance lies in the fact that the triangle is a potentially weak area in the anterior abdominal wall since it is not reinforced by the conjoint tendon. It is responsible for causing direct inguinal hernias.

What are the contents of the spermatic cord?
Apply the 'rule of 3s' (Table 1.2).

→ Testis

What is the blood supply to the testis?
The testis is supplied by the testicular artery which arises directly from the descending abdominal aorta approximately at the level of L2. The explanation lies in the fact that the testis develops high up on the posterior abdominal wall early in embryonic life. As it descends into the scrotum during development, the testis carries with it the same blood supply that it received whence it was positioned on the posterior abdominal wall (i.e. from the aorta).

What is the venous drainage of the testis?
There is asymmetry between the two sides. On the right side, the testis

Table 1.2
Contents of the spermatic cord: the rule of 3s

Three constituents: vas deferens (the round ligament is the female equivalent); lymphatics; obliterated processus vaginalis
Three nerves: genital branch of the genitofemoral nerve (motor to cremaster, sensory to cord); ilioinguinal nerve (within the inguinal canal but outside the spermatic cord); autonomics
Three arteries: testicular artery; artery to the vas (from the superior or inferior vesical artery); cremasteric artery (from the inferior epigastric artery).
Three veins: pampiniform plexus; vein from vas; cremasteric vein
Three fascial coverings: external spermatic fascia (derived from external oblique); cremasteric muscle and fascia (derived from internal oblique and transversus abdominis); internal spermatic fascia (derived from transversalis fascia)

drains by way of the pampiniform plexus into the inferior vena cava, but the left testis drains into the left renal vein. This may explain why varicoceles are more common on the left side.

What is the lymphatic drainage of the testis?

As a general rule regarding lymphatic drainage, superficial lymphatics (i.e. in subcutaneous tissues) tend to run with superficial veins, whereas deep lymphatics run with arteries. The testis thus drains lymph to the para-aortic set of lymph nodes, since the testicular artery arises from the aorta. The scrotum on the other hand drains to the inguinal group of lymph nodes. The testis, unlike the scrotum, never drains to the inguinal lymph nodes.

The clinical consequence of this is that a testicular carcinoma metastasises to the para-aortic group of lymph nodes and never results in inguinal lymphadenopathy, unless the scrotum is also involved. A scrotal carcinoma, on the other hand, causes inguinal lymphadenopathy.

What is the innervation of the testis?

The testis is supplied by T10 sympathetic nerves. The consequences of this are two-fold. First, it results in testicular pain (trauma, testicular torsion etc.) being referred to the umbilicus (T10 dermatome). Second, the ureters are also supplied by T10 sympathetics. Thus a renal calculus may refer pain down to the testis, as is seen in classical renal colic.

What layers does the surgeon traverse when operating on a testis?

- Skin
- Subcutaneous tissue (containing dartos muscle)
- Colles' fascia
- External spermatic fascia (external oblique)

- Cremaster muscle and fascia (internal oblique/transversus abdominis)
- Internal spermatic fascia (transversalis)
- Parietal layer of tunica vaginalis
- Visceral layer of tunica vaginalis
- Tunica albuginea of testis.

→ Ureters

What type of muscle do the ureters consist of?

The ureters are segmental muscular tubes, 25 cm long, composed of smooth (involuntary) muscle throughout their entire length.

What type of epithelium lines the ureters?

The ureters are lined by transitional epithelium (urothelium) throughout their length. Transitional epithelium is almost exclusively confined to the urinary tract of mammals where it is highly specialised to accommodate stretch and to withstand the toxicity of the urine.

How may the ureters be identified at surgery so as to prevent inadvertent ligation?

The ureter is characteristically a whitish, non-pulsatile cord, which shows peristaltic activity when gently pinched with forceps (i.e. it vermiculates).

What is the blood supply to the ureters?

Blood supply to the ureters, like the oesophagus, is segmental. The upper one-third is supplied by the renal arteries, the middle third from branches given off from the descending abdominal aorta, and the lower one-third is supplied by the superior and inferior vesical arteries. Blood supply to the middle third is the most tenuous. Consequently the middle third of the ureter is most vulnerable to postoperative ischaemia and stricture formation if blood supply to it is endangered by stripping the ureter clean of its surrounding tissue at surgery.

Where do the ureteric constrictions take place?

Along the course of the ureter are three narrowings that often form the site of obstruction in ureteric calculus disease:

- pelvi-ureteric junction
- where the ureter crosses the pelvic brim in the region of the bifurcation of the common iliac artery
- vesico-ureteric junction.

The vesico-ureteric junction is the point of narrowest calibre.

What is special about the way in which the ureters enter into the bladder?

In both sexes the ureters run obliquely through the bladder wall for 1–2 cm before reaching their orifices at the upper lateral angles of the trigone. This forms a flap valve preventing reflux of urine retrogradely back up the ureters. If this flap valve is congenitally deficient, vesico-ureteric reflux results.

➜   Hip joint

How is stability of the hip joint brought about?
As with all joints, stability is brought about by the way the various bones articulate with one another (through their incongruous surfaces) and through the various ligaments, tendons and muscles that surround the joint.

Stability is achieved largely as a result of the adaptation of the acetabulum and femoral head to one another, with a snug fit of the femoral head into the acetabulum, deepened by the labrum and further reinforced by three ligaments on the outside of the capsule (the iliofemoral, ischiofemoral and pubofemoral ligaments). The iliofemoral ligament (of Bigelow) is the strongest of the three ligaments. The short muscles of the gluteal region are important muscular stabilisers.

Since the hip is such a stable joint, it requires considerable force to become dislocated. When it does occur, it usually dislocates in the setting of a road traffic accident, where typically the hip joint dislocates posteriorly.

What are the important relations of the hip joint?
The hip joint lies deep to the pulsation of the femoral artery at the mid-inguinal point (half way between the anterior superior iliac spine and the symphysis pubis). Pain at this point may indicate pathology originating in the hip joint. Posterior to the hip lies the important sciatic nerve. Consequently, the sciatic nerve is at risk in a posterior surgical approach to the hip, or in a posterior dislocation.

What is the innervation of the hip joint?
The hip joint is innervated by the sciatic, femoral and obturator nerves (Hilton's law). The knee joint is also innervated by the same nerves. This may explain why hip pathology commonly refers pain to the knee. In a child who presents with a painful knee, always examine the ipsilateral hip joint, in addition to examining the knee, to avoid missing a diseased hip.

What is the blood supply to the femoral head, and what are the consequences of this?
The blood supply to the femoral head originates from three important sources:
- Most importantly, retinacular vessels run up from the trochanteric anastomosis and then along the neck of the femur to supply the major part of the head. The trochanteric anastomosis is formed by an anastomosis of the medial and lateral circumflex femoral arteries and the superior and inferior gluteal arteries.
- A second source is from the obturator artery in the ligamentum teres (round ligament). This is usually more important in children.

■ A third source is via the nutrient, or diaphyseal, artery of the femur, originating from the second perforating artery of the profunda femoris artery.

An intracapsular fractured neck of femur may disrupt the retinacular fibres and consequently disrupt the blood flow to the femoral head, resulting in avascular necrosis.

What is the Garden classification?

The Garden classification applies to all intracaspular fractures. Garden 1 and 2 fractures are undisplaced , while types 3 and 4 are displaced (Table 1.3).

Table 1.3
Garden classification of fractures

Grade	Type
I	Undisplaced, incomplete or impacted fracture
II	Undisplaced, complete fracture
III	Complete fracture with partial displacement
IV	Complete fracture with total displacement

How would you manage an intracapsular fracture?

Remember the adage 'one, two – screw; three, four – Austin-Moore'. Garden types 1 and 2 are generally treated by internal fixation with cannulated screws. Garden types 3 and 4 are generally treated with a hemiarthroplasty. The exception is the young patient with a type 3 or 4 where the aim is to try to save the hip – so open reduction and internal fixation is preferable in the first instance.

→ ## Shoulder joint

What type of joint is the shoulder joint?

The shoulder joint, like the hip joint, is a synovial joint of the ball and socket variety.

List the rotator cuff muscles, and what is their innervation?

There are four rotator cuff muscles; these may be remembered by the mnemonic SITS:
■ **s**upraspinatus – suprascapular nerve (C5, C6)
■ **i**nfraspinatus – suprascapular nerve (C5, C6)
■ **t**eres minor – axillary nerve (C5, C6)
■ **s**ubscapularis – upper and lower subscapular nerves (C5, C6).

What muscles attach to the coracoid process?

■ Coracobrachialis
■ Pectoralis minor
■ Short head of biceps.

What important nerve lies in close proximity to the shoulder joint?

It must never be forgotten that the axillary nerve lies in close proximity to the shoulder joint and the surgical neck of the humerus. Consequently, it is vulnerable to injury at the time of a shoulder dislocation, or while attempting to reduce the shoulder back into its normal position following a dislocation. It is therefore imperative (from both a clinical and medico-legal point of view) that the integrity of the axillary nerve is documented, both after seeing the patient who has a dislocated shoulder, but also following successful reduction.

→ Knee joint

What type of joint is the knee joint?

The knee joint is a synovial joint (the largest in the body), of the modified hinge variety.

Describe the cruciate ligaments of the knee joint.

The cruciate ligaments are two very strong ligaments that cross each other within the joint cavity, but are excluded from the synovial cavity by a covering of synovial membrane (they are therefore described as being intracapsular, but extrasynovial). They are crucial in the sense that they are essential for stability of the knee.

They are named anterior and posterior according to their tibial attachments. Thus the anterior cruciate ligament is attached to the anterior intercondylar area of the tibia and runs upwards, backwards and laterally to attach itself to the medial surface of the lateral femoral condyle. The anterior cruciate prevents anterior displacement of the tibia on the femur.

Backward displacement of the tibia on the femur is prevented by the stronger posterior cruciate ligament which runs from the posterior part of the tibial intercondylar area to the lateral aspect of the medial femoral condyle. The integrity of the latter is therefore important when walking down stairs or downhill. Tears of the anterior cruciate ligament are common in sports injuries; tears of the posterior cruciate ligament are rare since it is much stronger than the anterior cruciate.

Which bursae around the knee communicate with the joint?

Bursae are lubricating devices found wherever skin, muscle or tendon rubs against bone. There are approximately a dozen bursae related to the knee joint. The details are not important, only the salient points. For instance, the suprapatellar bursa communicates with the knee joint. An effusion of the knee may therefore extend some 3–4 finger breadths above the patella into the suprapatellar pouch. The prepatellar and infrapatellar bursae do not communicate with the knee joint, but may become inflamed causing a painful bursitis. Inflammation of the prepatellar bursa is known as housemaid's knee, whereas that of the infrapatellar bursa is called clergyman's knee.

Describe the menisci of the knee joint.

The menisci, or semilunar cartilages, are cresent-shaped laminae of fibrocartilage, the medial being larger and less curved than the lateral. They have an important role in:

- distributing the load by increasing the congruity of the articulation
- contributing to stability of the knee by their physical presence and by acting as providers of proprioceptive feedback
- acting as shock absorbers through a 'cushioning' effect
- probably assisting in lubrication.

The menisci are so effective that, if they are removed, the force taken by the articular hyaline cartilage during peak loading increases by about five-fold. Meniscectomy (removal of the menisci), or damage to the menisci, therefore exposes the articular hyaline cartilage to much greater forces than normal and evidence of degenerative osteoarthritis is seen in 75 per cent of patients 10 years after meniscectomy.

The menisci are liable to injury from twisting strains applied to a flexed weight-bearing knee. The medial meniscus is much less mobile than the lateral meniscus (because of its strong attachment to the medial collateral ligament of the knee joint) and therefore cannot as easily accommodate abnormal stresses placed upon it. This, in part, explains why medial meniscal tears are more common than lateral meniscal tears.

→ Femoral triangle

What are the boundaries of the femoral triangle?

The boundaries of the femoral triangle are the inguinal ligament superiorly, the medial border of adductor longus medially, and the medial border of sartorius laterally. The roof is fascia lata and the floor is made up of the following muscles: iliacus, psoas, pectineus, adductor longus.

What are the contents of the femoral triangle?

Use the mnemonic NAVY (lateral to medial):

- **N** = **n**erve (femoral) outside the femoral sheath
- **A** = **a**rtery (femoral) within the femoral sheath
- **V** = **v**ein (femoral) within the femoral sheath
- **Y** = **Y**-fronts (space most medially – deep inguinal lymph nodes).

What are the boundaries and contents of the femoral canal?

Within the femoral sheath lies the femoral artery, vein and a space most medially known as the femoral canal. The boundaries of the femoral canal are the femoral vein laterally, the lacunar ligament medially, the inguinal ligament anteriorly, and the pectineal ligament posteriorly.

Within the space of the femoral canal normally lies extraperitoneal fat and a lymph node which is often given its eponymous name, Cloquet's lymph node. Cloquet's lymph node drains the lower limb, perineum and anterior abdominal wall inferior to the umbilicus. It may be enlarged (as inguinal lymphadenopathy) in cases of carcinoma and infection at these sites.

The purpose of the femoral canal is to allow the laterally placed femoral vein to expand into it thereby encouraging venous return. However, a piece of bowel or omentum may extend down into the femoral space, causing a femoral hernia.

What is the surface anatomical landmark of the femoral artery?

The femoral artery lies at the mid-inguinal point (half way between the anterior superior iliac spine and symphysis pubis), not to be confused with the mid-point of the inguinal ligament (half way between the anterior superior iliac spine and the pubic tubercle) which is the surface marking of the deep inguinal ring.

This landmark can be used to assess the femoral pulse, but it also provides the clinician with a surface landmark for gaining access to the femoral artery for procedures such as coronary angioplasty and lower limb angiography and embolectomy.

What is the surface anatomical landmark of the adductor hiatus?

It is two-thirds the way along a line drawn from the anterior superior iliac spine to the adductor tubercle of the femur. Place your stethoscope at this point to auscultate for bruits in superficial femoral arterial disease in the claudicant patient.

→ Brachial plexus

What are the root values of the brachial plexus?

The brachial plexus has root values C5–C8 and T1. In 10 per cent of cases the brachial plexus may be either pre-fixed (C4–C8) or post-fixed (C6–T2).

Where are the different parts of the brachial plexus located?

See Fig. 1.5.

- *Roots*: exit their respective intervertebral foraminae between the scalenus anterior and medius muscles (interscalene space)
- *Trunks*: at the base of the posterior triangle of the neck, lying on the 1st rib posterior to the third part of the subclavian artery
- *Divisions*: behind the middle third of the clavicle
- *Cords*: in the axilla, in intimate relation to the second part of the axillary artery
- *Terminal branches*: in relation to the third part of the axillary artery.

The relation of the roots, trunks and divisions of the brachial plexus to the

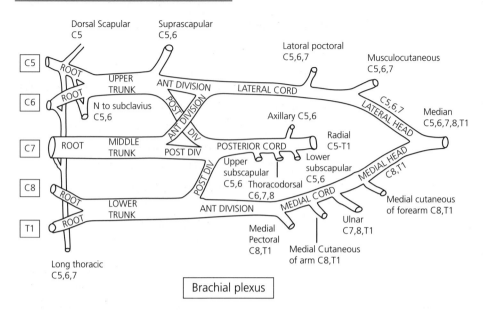

Brachial plexus

Figure 1.5 ● The brachial plexus.

scalene muscles, 1st rib and clavicle is important. Compression within a fixed space (the thoracic outlet) may lead to symptoms resulting from compression of the brachial plexus and/or nearby vascular structures (subclavian artery and vein). This is known as the thoracic outlet syndrome.

What are the main nerve derivatives of the 'cords' of the brachial plexus?

See Fig. 1.5.

- *Lateral cord*: musculocutaneous nerve
- *Medial cord*: ulnar nerve
- *Posterior cord*: radial nerve, axillary nerve
- *Medial and lateral cords*: median nerve.

What is the innervation of the serratus anterior muscle?

The serratus anterior muscle is innervated by the long thoracic nerve of Bell (C5, C6, C7). This may be remembered by the old aphorism 'C5, 6, 7 – bells of heaven'. Dennervation of the serratus muscle may result in winging of the scapula.

What are the two main patterns of injury to the brachial plexus?

There are two recognised types of brachial plexus palsy; both usually occur as a result of trauma or obstetric injury. The first follows injury to the upper roots of the brachial plexus (typically C5–C7) and is known as the Erb–Duchenne palsy. The arm typically lies in a waiter's tip position. The second follows injury to the lower roots of the brachial plexus (typically C8, T1) and is known as Klumpke's palsy. The hand in this case typically takes on the position of a 'clawed' hand.

→ Carpal tunnel

What is the carpal tunnel?

The carpal tunnel is a fibro-osseous tunnel situated on the flexor aspect of the proximal part of the hand and lying between the flexor retinaculum and the carpal bones. Compression of the median nerve within the carpal tunnel is known as carpal tunnel syndrome.

What does the carpal tunnel contain?

It contains the median nerve, together with 10 flexor tendons that include:

- four tendons of flexor digitorum superficialis
- four tendons of flexor digitorum profundus
- flexor carpi radialis tendon
- flexor pollicis longus tendon.

Note that the ulnar artery and nerve do not pass through the carpal tunnel, but instead pass superficial to the carpal tunnel in their own fibro-osseous tunnel, Guyon's canal. The ulnar nerve and artery are therefore unaffected in carpal tunnel syndrome.

Where does the flexor retinaculum attach?

The flexor retinaculum is attached to the tubercle of the scaphoid and pisiform proximally and the hook of the hamate and trapezium distally. Its function is to prevent bow-stringing of the flexor tendons at the wrist.

What muscles does the median nerve innervate in the hand?

The median nerve supplies four muscles in the hand, given by the mnemonic LOAF:

- **L** = **l**ateral two lumbricals
- **O** = **o**pponens pollicis
- **A** = **a**bductor pollicis brevis
- **F** = **f**lexor pollicis brevis.

Would you expect numbness over the thenar eminence in carpal tunnel syndrome?

No, because the palmar cutaneous branch of the median nerve is given off 5 cm proximal to the wrist and then passes superficial to the carpal tunnel.

How would you perform a carpal tunnel decompression?

Decompression can be performed:

- under general, regional or local anaesthesia
- open or endoscopic
- with or without a tourniquet.

First check that you are doing the right operation, for the right reasons (re-take history, re-examine as necessary and check nerve conduction studies (electrophysiology)). Fully inform the patient, obtain consent and mark the correct side.

- Position the arm extended and fully supinated on an arm board, with the hand held flat by a 'lead hand' retractor. Adopt standard preparation and drape to expose the whole hand.
- Begin your incision in line with the third web space distal to the distal wrist crease. Extend the incision proximal to the line of the first web space (thenar eminence). Ensure the skin incision is perpendicular to the skin. Protect the nerve with a Macdonald's elevator.
- Check that the flexor retinaculum is fully released (proximally and distally).
- Irrigate and ensure haemostasis.
- Close the wound with 3/0 nylon interrupted vertical mattress sutures. Apply a Mepore dressing and soft, non-constrictive hand bandage.
- Encourage elevation of the hand and early mobilisation, with analgesia.

What structures are at risk in a carpal tunnel decompression?

- Palmaris longus
- Palmar cutaneous branch of median nerve
- Recurrent motor branch of median nerve
- Superficial branch of the radial artery
- Ulnar artery and nerve
- Palmar arch (superficial and deep).

→ ## Anatomical snuffbox

What are the boundaries and contents of the anatomical snuffbox?

- *Base*: from proximal to distal – radial styloid, scaphoid, trapezium, base of 1st metacarpal
- *Roof*: skin; fascia
- *Medially* (ulnar side): extensor pollicis longus tendon
- *Laterally* (radial side): extensor pollicis brevis tendon; abductor pollicis longus tendon
- *Contents*: cephalic vein (beginning in its roof); terminal branches of radial nerve (supplying the overlying skin); radial artery (on its floor).

What is the surgical significance of the anatomical snuffbox?

Tenderness within the anatomical snuffbox may indicate a fractured scaphoid bone. This is important to recognise since X-rays are often unaltered in the early stages and, if left untreated, there is a high risk of avascular necrosis of the scaphoid (in fact the proximal scaphoid segment necroses since the scaphoid receives its blood supply from distal to proximal).

Tendonitis of the abductor pollicis longus and extensor pollicis brevis tendons may occur; this is known as DeQuervain's tenovaginitis stenosans.

The cephalic vein is almost invariably found in the region of the anatomical snuffbox. This is useful for gaining intravenous access.

→ ## Long saphenous vein

Describe the course of the long saphenous vein.

The long (great) saphenous vein, the longest vein in the body, begins as the upward continuation of the medial marginal vein of the foot. It courses upwards in front of the medial malleolus, in close proximity to the saphenous nerve, and runs up to lie a hand's breadth behind the medial border of the patella. It ends by passing through the cribriform fascia that covers the saphenous opening of the fascia lata. Here it joins the femoral vein at the saphenofemoral junction.

Like all superficial veins of the extremities, the long saphenous vein runs from superficial to deep and contains valves within its lumen. Both these factors prevent the reflux of blood and encourage venous return to the heart.

What is the surgical importance of knowing the anatomy of the long saphenous vein?

- Varicose veins and their surgical management
- Venous cut-down as an emergency
- Harvesting the vein as a graft in vascular and cardiothoracic surgery.

What is the course of the short saphenous vein?

The short (small) saphenous vein drains the lateral margin of the foot and lies with the sural nerve behind the lateral malleolus. It passes upwards in the subcutaneous fat to the midline of the calf and pierces the deep fascia to enter the popliteal vein at the saphenopopliteal junction.

How can you differentiate the long saphenous vein from the femoral vein at the saphenofemoral junction during varicose vein surgery, in order to prevent inadvertently ligating the wrong vessel?

- The long saphenous vein is more superficial than the femoral vein.
- The long saphenous vein has various tributaries in the region of the saphenous opening: superficial circumflex iliac vein, superficial epigastric vein, superficial and deep external pudendal veins.
- The femoral vein at this level receives only the long saphenous vein itself.

Which nerves may be injured in varicose vein surgery?

- *Long* saphenous vein surgery: the saphenous nerve (branch of the femoral nerve)
- *Short* saphenous vein surgery: the sural nerve.

Surgical pathology

Introduction

→ Structuring your answers in pathology

- Define
- Classify
- Amplify.

→ Classifications

- Congenital versus acquired
- Benign versus malignant
- Malignancies: primary versus secondary (metastatic)
- Aetiology: use the 'surgical sieve' – i.e. 'INVITED MD' (congenital/genetic + infections, neoplasia, vascular, inflammatory, trauma, endocrine, degenerative, metabolic, drugs and toxins + immune/autoimmune + idiopathic)
- Complications: general/systemic versus specific/local
- Complications: immediate, early or late
- Effects of tumours: locally invasive versus distant effects (metastatic and non-metastatic/paraneoplastic).

→ College favourites

- Inflammation: acute and chronic: inflammatory bowel disease
- Wound healing: primary; secondary intention; factors affecting wound healing
- Neoplasia: metaplasia; dysplasia; invasion; metastasis
- Staging and grading: TNM classification; Dukes' classification
- Thrombus; embolus; Virchow's triad
- Referral to Coroner
- Infections: tuberculosis/mycobacteria; HIV etc.
- Fistulae; sinuses; abscess
- Weird and wonderful: amyloidosis; pathology specimen pots.

Neoplasia

B&L   For further reading see *Bailey and Love*, Chapter 7

→ Neoplasms

What is a neoplasm?
It is an abnormal mass of tissue, the growth of which:

- is uncoordinated
- exceeds that of normal tissues
- persists in the same excessive manner after cessation of the stimulus that evoked the change (Willis).

How may neoplasms be classified?

They are best divided into:

- neoplastic growth disorders
- non-neoplastic growth disorders (hyperplasia, hypertrophy, hamartoma, metaplasia, dysplasia).

Neoplasms can also be classified as *benign* or *malignant*. Malignant neoplasms can be further classified as *primary* or *secondary* (metastatic).

How may neoplasms be classified according to cell type of origin (histogenesis)?

One cell type:

- Epithelial: papilloma, adenoma, carcinoma
- Mensenchymal: fibroma, lipoma, sarcoma
- Lymphoma.

More than one cell type from one germ layer:

- Pleomorphic adenoma, fibroadenoma breast, Wilms' tumour.

More than one cell type from more than one germ layer:

- Teratomas (may be benign or malignant).

How may neoplasms be classified according to behaviour?

Classification is into benign versus malignant (Table 2.1).

Table 2.1
Classification of neoplasms

Benign	Malignant
Non-invasive **No metastasis**	**Invasive** **Capable of metastasis**
Resembles tissue of origin (well differentiated)	Variable resemblance to tissue of origin
Slowly growing	Rapidly growing
Normal nuclear morphology	Abnormal nuclear morphology
Well circumscribed (pseudocapsule)	Irregular border
Rare necrosis/ulceration	Common necrosis/ulceration

→ Hyperplasia

What is hyperplasia? Give some examples.

Hyperplasia is an increase in size of an organ or tissue through an increase in the *number* of cells. The cells mature to normal size and morphology.

- Physiological examples: breast; thyroid in pregnancy
- Pathological examples: overstimulation – adrenals in Cushing's; Graves' disease.

→ Hypertrophy

What is hypertrophy? Give some examples.
Hypertrophy is an increase in size of an organ or tissue through an increase in the *size* of cells. There are the same number of cells which mature to normal morphology.
- Physiological examples: skeletal muscle with exercise; uterus in pregnancy
- Pathological example: cardiomyopathy.

→ Hamartomas

What is a hamartoma? Give some examples.
A hamartoma is a tumour-like malformation composed of a haphazard arrangement of the different amounts of tissues normally found at that site. It grows under normal growth controls of the body.
- Examples: Peutz–Jegher's polyps of bowel; haemangiomas.

→ Metaplasia

What is metaplasia, and what is its significance?
Metaplasia is a *reversible* replacement of one fully differentiated cell type with another differentiated cell type. It represents an adaptive change, in response to injury, irritation or altered cell function.
- There is greater susceptibility to malignant transformation
- Misdiagnosis will lead to overtreatment.

Give four examples of metaplasia.
- Barrett's oesophagus secondary to reflux oesophagitis – change from stratified squamous to glandular, columnar type epithelium
- Bronchus secondary to cigarette smoking – change from normal respiratory epithelium which is pseudostratified ciliated columnar to stratified squamous
- Transformation zone of the cervix secondary to human papilloma virus (HPV) – change from normal columnar endocervical epithelium to stratified squamous
- Carcinoma of the bladder secondary to chronic irritation – calculi/schistosomes.

→ Dysplasia

What is dysplasia?
Dysplasia is disordered cellular development characterised by increased mitosis and pleomorphism BUT without the ability to invade through the basement membrane and metastasise to distant sites.
- Severe dysplasia = carcinoma-in-situ.

→ Carcinomas and sarcomas

What are carcinomas and sarcomas?
- A carcinoma is a malignant tumour of epithelial cells.
- A sarcoma is a malignant tumour of connective tissue.

How do carcinomas and sarcomas typically spread?
As a general rule, carcinomas typically spread via the lymphatic route; sarcomas typically spread by the haematogenous route. However, there are exceptions to this rule; e.g. follicular thyroid carcinomas spread via the bloodstream to bone.

What makes a tumour malignant?
The key features of malignancy are:
- invasion through the basement membrane
- the ability to metastasise to distant sites.

→ Metastasis and routes of tumour spread

What is a metastasis?
A metastasis is the survival and growth of cells that have migrated or have otherwise been transferred from a malignant tumour to a site or sites distant from the primary.

What are the routes by which tumours spread?
- Local invasion
- Lymph – most carcinomas
- Blood – sarcomas and follicular carcinoma of thyroid
- Transcoelomic – carcinoma of stomach, ovary, colon and pancreas; pseudomyxoma peritonei
- Cerebrospinal fluid – CNS tumours (gliomatosis cerebri)
- Perineural – adenoid cystic carcinoma of the parotid gland
- Iatrogenic – implantation/seeding during surgery.

Which tumours typically spread to bone?
Bone is a favoured site of metastasis from carcinoma of the breast, bronchus, thyroid, kidney and prostate, and myeloma.

→ Cytological and histological features of malignancy

B&L For further reading see *Bailey and Love*, Chapter 12.

What are the cytological and histological features of malignancy?

Cytological features
- Hyperchromatism (dark-staining nuclei because of increased amounts of DNA)
- Pleomorphism (variance of size and shape of tumour cells and nuclei)

Inapp
activ
cellular

B&L For further reading see *Bailey and Love*, pp. 823–826.

What is multiple endocrine neoplasia (MEN)?

MEN is a group of related conditions, inherited as autosomal dominant traits, characterised by hyperplasias and/or neoplasms of several endocrine organs. The genetic defect in MEN 1 has been linked to a novel gene on chromosome 11 (*MENIN* gene). MEN 2 is clinically and genetically distinct from MEN 1 and has been linked to mutations in the RET proto-oncogene located on chromosome 10.

MEN 1 = 3Ps

- Pituitary adenomas (prolactinomas most commonly)
- Pancreatic islet cell tumours (gastrinomas most commonly)
- Parathyroids (hyperplasia).

MEN 2a

- Medullary thyroid carcinoma
- Phaeochromocytoma
- Parathyroid hyperplasia.

MEN 2b

- Medullary thyroid carcinoma
- Phaeochromocytoma
- Marfanoid-type body habitus
- Mucosal neuromatosis.

Inflammation

➜ Acute inflammation

What is acute inflammation?

Acute inflammation is a stereotypical response to tissue injury. It is characterised by:

- heat, pain, redness, swelling ('calor, dolor, rubor, tumor')
- +/− functio laesa (loss of function)
- +/− fluor (secretion).

Define the stages of inflammation.

- Vasodilatation
- Increased vascular permeability
- Diapedesis
- Phagocytosis
- Resolution or progression to chronic inflammation.

Name some chemical mediators that participate in acute inflammation.

- Vasoactive amines (histamine, 5-HT/serotonin)
- Kinin system (bradykinin)
- Complement cascade (C3a, C5a)

- Coagulation cascade and fibrinolytic system
- Arachidonic acid metabolites (leukotrienes, prostaglandins, thromboxane A2)
- Cytokines (interleukins, TNFα, TGFβ etc.).

What are the possible outcomes of acute inflammation?
- Resolution
- Progression to chronic inflammation
- Organisation and repair culminating in scar formation
- Death (meningitis is a good example)
- Abscess formation (this may spontaneously drain to a surface by means of a sinus or fistula).

→ Chronic inflammation

What is chronic inflammation? Give some examples of its causes.
Chronic inflammation is defined by the cell types present (macrophages, lymphocytes). It typically has a longer time course than acute inflammation. Causes include:
- persistent infection that evades host defence mechanisms (tuberculosis, syphilis, leprosy, H. pylori)
- endogenous injurious agent (acid in stomach in peptic ulcer disease)
- persistent/non-degradable toxin (silica dust, asbestos, lipids in arterial walls – arteriosclerosis)
- host attacks on components of self (autoimmune diseases – rheumatoid arthritis, Hashimoto's)
- host resistance suppressed (immunodeficiency states – HIV, malnutrition, prolonged steroid use)
- unknown/idiopathic (sarcoidosis, inflammatory bowel disease).

What are the pathological consequences of chronic inflammation?
- Tissue destruction and scarring
- Malignant transformation
- Amyloidosis.

→ Wound healing

B&L **For further reading see *Bailey and Love*, Chapter 3.**

What is wound healing, and how may it be classified?
Wound healing is the process by which tissue restoration of structure and function occurs, with restitution of tissue integrity and tensile strength. Wound healing can be classified into healing by:
- primary intention
- secondary intention (granulation)
- delayed primary (tertiary) intention.

Wounds can heal by resolution (no scar formation) or by organisation and repair, which invariably results in scar tissue.

Figure 2.2 ●
Delayed healing
relating to infection
in a patient on
high-dose steroids.
(Bailey and Love,
Figure 4.2, p. 34.)

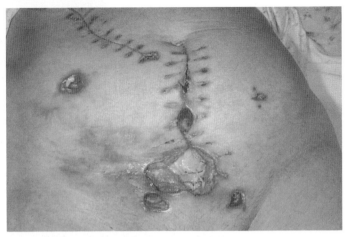

What are the stages of wound healing?
- Haemostasis/coagulation
- Acute inflammation
- Formation of granulation tissue (endothelial cells, fibroblasts, macrophages)
- Angiogenesis
- Epithelialisation, fibroplasia, wound contraction (myofibroblasts)
- Maturation and remodelling.

What factors affect wound healing?
- *Local factors*: poor blood supply; haematoma; infection (Fig. 2.2); foreign bodies; surgical technique (excessive wound tension, type of suture material); radiotherapy
- *General/systemic factors*: diabetes mellitus; steroids; immunodeficiency; heart failure; renal failure; liver failure; hypoxia; malnutrition; chemotherapy; malignancy.

What is the key difference between hypertrophic and keloid scarring?
A hypertrophic scar is confined to the wound margins. Such scars often occur across flexor surfaces and skin creases. A keloid scar (Greek *kele* = claw + *eidos* = like) extends beyond the wound margins. Keloid scars are more common in patients of Black and Hispanic descent and characteristically occur in the earlobe, chin, neck, shoulder, chest and deltoid regions (Fig. 2.3).

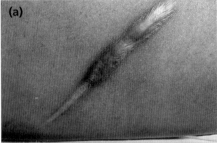

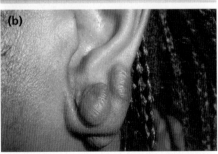

Figure 2.3 ● (a) Hypertrophic scar after a knife wound. It is raised and stretched, but confined to the boundary of the initial incision. (b) Keloid scar, following an ear-piercing, which is dumbbell shaped, in three dimensions. This became keloid several years after the piercing. (Bailey and Love, Figures 39.9a and 39.9c, p. 599.)

→ Common definitions

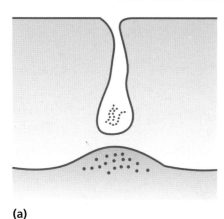

(a)

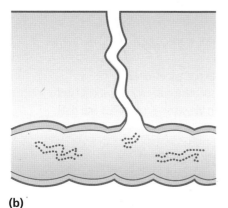

(b)

Figure 2.4 ● Sinus and fistula, both usually arise from a preceding abcess. (a) A blind track, in this case a pilonidal abscess. (b) A track connecting two epithelium-lined surfaces, in this case a colocutaneous fistula from colon to skin. (Bailey and Love, Figures 39.4a and 39.4b, p. 596.)

What is an abscess?
An abscess is a localised collection of pus surrounded by granulation tissue/fibrous tissue.

What is pus?
Pus is a collection of neutrophils, together with dead and dying micro-organisms.

What is a sinus, and how does it differ from a fistula?
A sinus is a blind-ending track lined by granulation tissue. A fistula is an abnormal communication between two epithelial surfaces (or endothelial surfaces – e.g. arteriovenous fistula) (Fig. 2.4). The commonest fistula is an ear-piercing.

What is a stoma?
A stoma is a surgical opening into a hollow viscus. It can be classified by anatomical site, output (colostomy, ileostomy, urostomy, tracheostomy, gastrostomy etc.), indication (temporary versus permanent), or the number of openings (end versus loop).

→ Fistulae

How may fistulae be classified?
■ Congenital (e.g. tracheo-oesophageal fistula) versus acquired
■ Aetiology (infections, inflammation, malignancy, radiotherapy)
■ Internal versus external
■ Simple versus complex
■ Anatomy: by site (e.g. entero-enteric, entero-cutaneous, colo-vaginal, vesico-colic)
■ Physiology: high-output (>500 mL/day) versus low-output.

What factors prevent an intestinal fistula from healing spontaneously?

- Distal obstruction
- Malignancy
- Foreign body
- Associated undrained infection
- Radiation injury to tissues
- Underlying inflammatory condition (e.g. Crohn's)
- Mucocutaneous continuity
- High output
- Malnutrition.

How are fistulae managed?

The mnemonic SNAP is useful:

- **S** = **s**epsis control (Fig. 2.5)
- **N** = **n**utritional support
- **A** = **a**natomical assessment + **a**dequate fluid and electrolyte replacement
- **P** = **p**lan + **p**rotect skin to prevent excoriation.

Sixty per cent should close spontaneously within 1 month with conservative measures when the sepsis is controlled and distal obstruction has been relieved.

→ Inflammatory bowel disease

Inflammatory bowel disease (IBD) is a good example of chronic inflammation. It can be classified as:

- Crohn's disease
- ulcerative colitis
- indeterminate colitis.

Figure 2.5 ● Major wound infection and delayed healing presenting as a faecal fistula in a patient with Crohn's disease. (Bailey and Love, Figure 4.1, p. 34.)

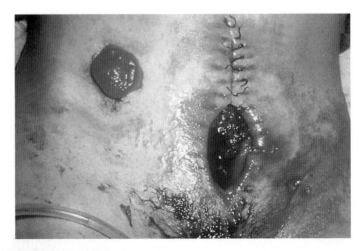

What are the macroscopic and microscopic differences between Crohn's disease and ulcerative colitis?

See Table 2.3.

Table 2.3
Comparison of Crohn's disease and ulcerative colitis

Crohn's	Ulcerative colitis
Anywhere in the GI tract	Rectum
Skip lesions	Confined to colon
Rectal sparing	Contiguous disease
Full thickness/transmural	+/– backwash ileitis
Fat wrapping	Mucosal disease
Deep fissures	Pseudopolyps
Fistulae, sinuses	No granulomas
Strictures → obstruction	Crypt abscesses (UC > CD)
Non-caseating granulomas (~60%)	'Lead pipe' colon
'Cobblestone' mucosa	Dysplasia

What are the extra-intestinal manifestations of IBD?

■ Integument: clubbing; erythema nodosum; pyoderma gangrenosum; aphthous ulcers
■ Eyes: conjunctivitis; episcleritis; scleritis; anterior uveitis
■ Liver and biliary tree: fatty liver; chronic active hepatitis; cirrhosis; gallstones; primary sclerosing cholangitis; cholangiocarcinoma
■ Renal tract: calculi
■ Joints: peripheral arthopathy; sacroiliitis; ankylosing spondylitis
■ Amyloidosis.

→ ## Granulomas

What is a granuloma? Give some examples.

A granuloma is a focal area of chronic inflammation. It consists of a microscopic aggregation of activated macrophages that are transformed into epithelium-like cells, surrounded by a collar of mononuclear leucocytes, principally lymphocytes and plasma cells.

Granulomas can be classified into caseating (e.g. tuberculosis) versus non-caseating (sarcoid, Wegener's granulomatosis, Crohn's, primary biliary cirrhosis).

■ *Infections:* TB; leprosy; syphilis; actinomycosis
■ *Inflammation:* sarcoidosis; Crohn's; primary biliary cirrhosis; Wegener's granulomatosis
■ *Foreign bodies:* beryllium; silicon; talc; sutures
■ *Malignancy:* Hodgkin's disease.

Other topics commonly asked about

→ Aneurysms

What is an aneurysm?
An aneurysm is an abnormal, permanent, localised dilatation of a blood vessel, to 1.5–2 times its normal diameter (Fig. 2.6).

How are aneurysms classified?
- Aetiology (e.g. atherosclerotic, inflammatory)
- Congenital versus acquired
- True versus false (pseudoaneurysm)
- Site (e.g. thoracic, abdominal, intracranial)
- Size (e.g. giant aneurysms, berry)
- Shape (e.g. fusiform, saccular, dissecting).

Figure 2.6 ● Operative appearance of a large, non-ruptured infrarenal abdominal aortic aneurysm. (Bailey and Love, Figure 53.45, p. 921.)

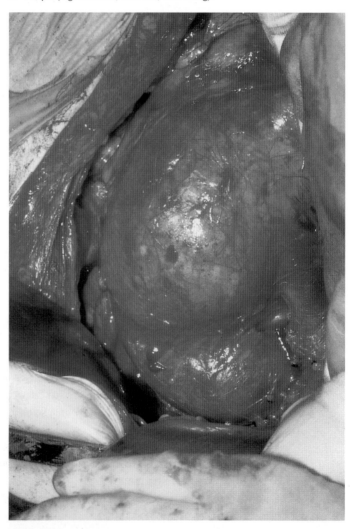

What are the complications of aneurysms?

- Rupture
- Thrombosis
- Embolism
- Local compressive effects
- Infection (mycotic)
- Fistula (e.g. aorto-enteric fistula).

→ Polyps

What is a polyp? Name some different types.

A polyp is a pedunculated mass of tissue arising from an epithelial surface. Polyps can be classified into non-neoplastic and neoplastic types:

- Non-neoplastic polyps: hyperplastic (also known as metaplastic); hamartomatous; inflammatory pseudopolyps; lymphoid hyperplasia
- Neoplastic polyps: tubular; tubulo-villous; villous.

In terms of frequency: tubular (65–80 per cent) > tubulo-villous (10–25 per cent) > villous (5–10 per cent). In terms of malignant potential: villous (40 per cent risk of harbouring cancer) > tubulo-villous (22 per cent) > tubular (5 per cent).

What complications might polyps undergo?

- Malignant transformation
- Ulceration
- Bleeding
- Infection
- Intussusception
- Protein and potassium loss.

→ Diverticula

What are diverticula, and how are they classified?

A diverticulum is an abnormal outpouching of a hollow viscus into the surrounding tissues. Diverticula can be classified as follows:
Aetiology:

- Congenital (Meckel's) versus acquired
- Pulsion versus traction*

Location:

- Site (oesophagus – e.g. Zenker's diverticulum; small intestine, large intestine)
- Mesenteric (small intestine) versus anti-mesenteric location (Meckel's)

Architecture:

- True (Meckel's) versus false (sigmoid colon, pharyngeal pouch).

*Most diverticula are of the pulsion variety. Traction diverticula are much less common and are mostly a consequence of fibrotic healing in lymph nodes secondary to chronic granulomatous disease exerting traction on the neighbouring bowel wall.

What complications might a diverticulum undergo?

- Perforation
- Inflammation +/− infection
- Bleeding
- Fistulae
- Strictures
- Malignancy (e.g. bladder diverticula).

→ ## Thrombosis and emboli

What are the differences between a clot, a thrombus and an embolus?

A thrombus is defined as solid material formed from the constituents of blood in flowing blood. When formed in stationary blood, it is a clot. An embolus is defined as an abnormal mass of undissolved material that is carried in the bloodstream from one place to another.

What causes a thrombus?

Virchow's triad:

See Fig. 2.7.

- damage to a vessel wall
- alterations in blood flow
- alterations in the constituents of the blood.

Figure 2.7 ●
Virchow's triad.

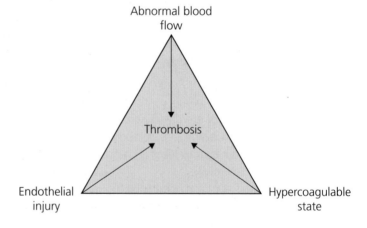

What are the different types of emboli?

An embolus can be solid, liquid or gas:

- a thrombus
- fat
- air
- atheromatous material
- amniotic fluid
- tumour cells
- foreign material (e.g. broken cannula).

→ Atherosclerosis

What is atherosclerosis, and how does it arise?

Atherosclerosis is a chronic inflammatory process and is a disease of the tunica intima. It is reversible upon removing the injurious agent – hence the importance of risk factor modification and primary prevention strategies.

The 'response to injury' hypothesis seems most plausible in explaining the underlying pathogenesis. It explains how the biggest risk factors exert their influence (tobacco toxins, hypertension and turbulent blood flow, lipids, glycosylated haemoglobin in diabetes mellitus), and why risk factor modification is so successful in modifying the disease process.

What are the complications of atherosclerosis?

- Distal ischaemia
- Vessel occlusion
- Plaque ulceration, rupture
- Thrombosis
- Haemorrhaging into a plaque
- Embolism (lipid or thrombus)
- Calcification
- Aneurysm formation.

→ Necrosis and apoptosis

What is necrosis? What are the different types?

Necrosis is defined as abnormal tissue death during life. Necrosis is always pathological and is accompanied by inflammation. Groups of cells are involved and undergo swelling and lysis. Necrotic cells are phagocytosed by inflammatory cells. There are several different types of necrosis.

- *Coagulative* (structured) necrosis is the most common form. It results from interruption of blood supply. Tissue architecture is preserved. Coagulative necrosis is seen in organs supplied by end arteries, such as kidney, heart, liver and spleen.
- *Liquefactive* (colliquative) necrosis occurs in tissues rich in lipid where lysosomal enzymes denature the fat and cause liquefaction of the tissue. This characteristically occurs in the brain.
- *Caseous* (unstructured) necrosis has the gross appearance of soft, cheesy friable material. Tissue architecture is destroyed. It is commonly seen in tuberculosis.
- *Fat* necrosis can occur following direct trauma (e.g. in breast) or enzymatic lipolysis (e.g. pancreatitis).
- *Fibrinoid* necrosis is seen in the walls of arteries that are subjected to high pressures, as in malignant hypertension. The muscular wall undergoes necrosis and is associated with deposition of fibrin.
- *Gangrenous* necrosis is irreversible tissue death characterised by putrefaction. It may be wet, dry or gaseous. The tissues appear green or black because of breakdown of haemoglobin.

Table 2.4
Comparison of apoptosis and necrosis

Apoptosis	Necrosis
Energy dependent (active)	Energy independent
Internally programmed (suicide)	Response to external injury
Affects single cells	Affects groups of cells
No accompanying inflammation	Accompanied by inflammation
Physiological or pathological	Always pathological
Plasma membrane remains intact	Loss of plasma membrane integrity
Cell shrinkage, fragmentation and formation of apoptotic bodies	Cell swelling and lysis

What is the difference between apoptosis and necrosis?
See Table 2.4.

→ ## Hypersensitivity reactions

What are hypersensitivity reactions?
A hypersensitivity reaction is a condition in which undesirable tissue damage follows the development of humeral or cell-mediated immunity. It represents an exaggerated response of the host's immune system to a particular stimulus.

How may hypersensitivity reactions be classified?
Hypersensitivity reactions can be distinguished according to Gell and Coombs' classification (Table 2.5). The original description by Gell and Coombs was based on four classes, with a fifth class being added later.

→ ## Leg ulcers

What is an ulcer? Give some examples of leg ulcers.
An ulcer is a break in an epithelial surface. The commonest leg ulcers are:
- venous (70 per cent of cases)
- arterial
- neuropathic.

Other causes include:
- infection (e.g. tuberculosis, leprosy, syphilis)
- malignancy (e.g. squamous or basal cell carcinoma, melanoma, Marjolin's, Kaposi's sarcoma)
- haematological condition (e.g. haemolytic anaemias, sickle cell, polycythaemia rubra vera, thalassaemia)
- vasculitides (e.g. rheumatoid arthritis, polyarteritis nodosa)
- metabolic (e.g. pyoderma gangrenosum)
- trauma (e.g. lacerations, burns, radiation, self-inflicted)
- iatrogenic (e.g. over-tight bandaging, ill-fitting plaster cast)
- idiopathic.

Table 2.5
Gell and Coombs' classification of hypersensitivity reactions

Type	Features
I	Mast cell degranulation mediated by preformed IgE bound to mast cells Immediate (within minutes) Anaphylaxis Atopic allergies
II	Antibodies directed towards antigens present on the surface of cells or tissue components Humoral antibodies participate directly in injuring cells by predisposing them to phagocytosis or lysis Good examples are transfusion reactions, autoimmune haemolytic anaemia and Goodpasture's syndrome Initiates within several hours
III	Formation of antibody–antigen complexes (immune complex mediated) Good examples are the Arthus reaction, serum sickness, and SLE Initiates in several hours
IV	Delayed type of hypersensitivity Cell-mediated T-lymphocytes involved Granulomatous conditions Contact dermatitis Initiation time is 24–72 hours
V	Due to the formation of stimulatory autoantibodies in autoimmune conditions such as Graves' disease and myasthenia gravis

→ # Tumour markers

What is a tumour marker?
A tumour marker is a substance reliably found in the circulation of a patient with neoplasia which is directly related to the presence of the neoplasm, disappears when the neoplasm is treated, and reappears when the neoplasm recurs.

Give some examples of tumour markers.
- Hormones (e.g. βHCG, calcitonin)
- Enzymes (e.g. prostate-specific antigen, placental alanine aminotransferase, lactate dehydrogenase)
- Oncofetal antigens (e.g. α-fetoprotein, carcinoembryonic antigen, CA-125, CA19-9)
- Serum and tissue proteins (e.g. thyroglobulin).

What are the possible uses of tumour markers?
- Diagnostic purposes
- Prognostic information (tumour load)
- Monitoring response to treatment
- Surveillance to detect recurrence
- Screening.

■ Is expensive
■ Potential for spread of malignant cells
■ May alter morphology of lesion for subsequent imaging.

→ ## Referral to the Coroner

When would you refer a death to the Coroner?

A death should be referred to the Coroner if:

■ a doctor has not attended the deceased within 14 days of death or in terminal illness
■ the cause is unknown
■ it was sudden (including all within 24 hours of hospital admission)
■ it occurred during an operation or before recovery from the effects of an anaesthetic
■ it might be due to an accident (whenever it occurred)
■ it might be due to self-neglect or neglect by others
■ it was violent, unnatural or suspicious
■ it might be due to suicide
■ it might be due to an abortion
■ it might be due to an industrial disease or related to the deceased's employment
■ it occurred during or shortly after detention in police or prison custody.

Applied surgical science

The operating room

B&L   For further reading see *Bailey and Love*, Chapter 15.

How would you construct and organise the ideal operating room?

- Locate it near to the Intensive Care, Accident and Emergency and Radiology departments.
- Separate it from the main hospital traffic.
- A single floor should be reserved for the operating suites.
- To reduce solar heat gain or loss, the operating suites should be located in the lower hospital levels.
- Streams of clean and dirty traffic should be separated to avoid contamination.
- There should be a transfer and changeover area at the entry and exit points.
- There should be protective areas: recovery, changing room and offices.
- There should be at least three zones: clean, sterile and disposal.
  - *Clean zone:* scrub rooms, gowning areas, exit lobby, rest areas and sterile stores.
  - *Sterile zone:* the operating theatre and sterile preparation rooms.
  - *Disposal zone:* the least clean area – disposal sluice or sink rooms.
- Hospital staff should move from one clean area to another without having to pass through unprotected or traffic areas.
- Airflow direction should be from the clean to less clean areas. There should be no airflow between theatre suites.
- Heating, air-conditioning and ventilation should allow for comfortable working conditions.
- The operating suites should have good lighting (artificial and natural).
  - General lighting of theatres should be provided by fluorescent tubes or filament lamps producing illumination with little or no glare.
  - The main operating lights are complemented by direct light from several angles to reduce shadows.
- Electricity should be maintained with emergency support (supplementary generator) in case of power failure. The main voltage is between 220 and 240 V, 50 Hz. Switches and sockets should be spark-free.
- A clean environment is important.
  - Smooth surfaces are easily washable.
  - Joins between walls, ceiling and floors should be curved to reduce dirt collection.
  - Floors should be impervious with antistatic properties. They should be easy to wash and may be made of rubber or vinyl.
- The colour of the operating suites should be pale-blue, grey or green in order to be less tiring on the eyes.

In the operating theatre, what is the goal of ventilation?

- Comfort to all hospital staff
- Removal of anaesthetic gas
- Air that is free of pathological organisms.

What types of ventilation are used in operating rooms?

Ventilation should allow air to pass through a steam humidifier, resulting in 50–60 per cent relative humidity. Combined with background heating, the ventilation system can be used to adjust the temperature in the operating suites to between 18.5° and 22°C.

Turbulent air flow system

Positive pressure is used to prevent dirty air entering the sterile operating suites. The air pressure should be higher than in surrounding areas. Air is drawn by fans via filters and humidified into the operating areas.

Laminar flow displacement system

The high-impact and high-exhaust system was first introduced by Charnley. Air flows at a unidirectional horizontal velocity and passes through filters to remove contamination. Positive pressurisation is used. The displaced air is not recycled but moves away from the operating site.

Surgical diathermy

What is diathermy?

Diathermy (electrocoagulation) is the passage of high-frequency alternating current (AC) to produce a localised heating effect, resulting in local tissue destruction, sealing of blood vessels and the arrest of bleeding.

What are the types of diathermy?

Monopolar (unipolar)

The current flows from a current generator to a small active electrode held by the operating surgeon. The tip of the electrode represents a point of high current density where the heat is generated. The current then flows through the patient and ends at a second electrode, the diathermy plate.

Bipolar

The current passes down one arm of the forceps, through structures between the forceps tips and then returns through the other arm of the forceps. A loop is created.

What is the surface area of the monopolar diathermy plate?

The surface area is at least 70 cm².

What are the diathermy modes?

- *Cutting:* In this (continuous) mode, an electrical arc is used to cut tissues and cauterise the divided surface. Cell water is vaporised, resulting in tissue destruction.
- *Coagulation:* In this (fulguration) mode, a pulsed high-intensity output passes through the tissues, causing tissue desiccation and sealing of blood vessels.
- *Blend:* This is a mixture of the cutting and coagulation modes.

What are the potential complications of diathermy?

Burns and thermal injury are the major complications of diathermy use, resulting from:

- incorrect application of the diathermy plate
- patient in contact with earth metals
- poor technique
- capacitance coupling (inductive coupling occurs when an electrode is inside an insulator with a further conductor outside – laparoscopic ports) (Fig 5.3)
- direct coupling of instruments (Fig. 3.1)
- fire and explosion as a result of pooling of alcohol-based skin preparations
- explosion of bowel
- carcinogenic surgical smoke.

Can diathermy be used in patients with pacemakers?

There is a potential risk of arrhythmias or cardiac damage when diathermy is used in patients with implanted or external pacemakers. The risk is increased if the pacemaker and its connections are in the direct pathway between the active electrode and the plate.

Diathermy should be avoided in patients with electronic implants. If diathermy is required, bipolar diathermy should be used. The plate and active electrode should be placed away from the thorax. Coagulation should be used in short bursts. External pacing should be available in case of cardiac dysfunction.

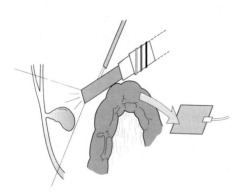

Figure 3.1 ● Direct coupling between bowel and laparoscope, which is touching the activated probe. (Bailey and Love, Figure 19.10, p. 254.)

Who is responsible for the use and complications of diathermy in the operating theatre?

The operating surgeon is responsible.

Uses of the stethoscope

What are the uses of the stethoscope in surgery?

Preoperative assessment of organ systems
- Cardiovascular conditions (e.g. murmurs)
- Blood pressure measurement
- Vascular conditions (e.g. carotid and renal bruits, ankle–brachial pressure index – ABPI)
- Respiratory conditions (e.g. pneumonia)
- Gastrointestinal conditions (e.g. obstruction, ileus)
- Neurological conditions (e.g. AV fistula).

Operative
Confirm placement of the endotracheal tube.

Postoperative assessment of organ systems
- Cardiovascular conditions (e.g. pulmonary oedema)
- Blood pressure measurement
- Respiratory conditions (e.g. pneumonia, atelectasis)
- Gastrointestinal conditions (e.g. obstruction, ileus, nasogastric tube placement).

Stomas

B&L   For further reading see *Bailey and Love*, pp.1185–1187.

What is a stoma?
In medicine, a stoma is an opening, either natural or surgically created, which connects a portion of a cavity to another area (Fig. 3.2).

A natural stoma is any opening in the body, such as the mouth. Any hollow organ can be manipulated into an artificial stoma. Surgical procedures that create stomas begin with a prefix denoting the organ, or area, being operated on and end with the suffix '-ostomy'.

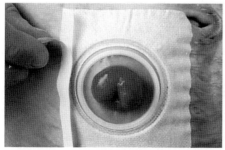

What are the uses of a stoma?
Remember the mnemonic FLED:
- **F** = **f**eeding
- **L** = **l**avage
- **E** = **e**xteriorisation
- **D** = **d**ecompression, **d**iversion and **d**rainage.

Figure 3.2 ● The usual long-term backing ('stomahesive') and flange, onto which the bag is being placed. (Bailey and Love, Figure 65.51a, p. 1186.)

What are the types of stoma?

- Temporary versus permanent
- End versus loop
- Based on anatomical location (tracheostomy, pharyngostomy, oesophagostomy, gastrostomy, duodenostomy, jejunostomy, ileostomy, colostomy, caecostomy, urostomy, nephrostomy).

How is an abdominal stoma site chosen?

Preoperatively, the stoma site is marked on the skin while the patient is standing and sitting. The selected site should be away from the potential surgical incision, umbilicus and bony points. A stoma nurse should be involved in the patient's overall care.

Intraoperatively, a stoma should be created without tension, with viable bowel and with an adequate vascular supply.

What are the potential complications of stomas?

Immediate:

- Bleeding
- Ischaemia
- Necrosis.

Early:

- High output
- Obstruction
- Retraction.

Late:

- Obstruction
- Prolapse
- Retraction
- Stenosis
- Parastomal hernia
- Skin excoriation and hypersensitivity
- Electrolyte disturbance
- Fistula formation
- Stone (renal and gall) formation
- Psychological and psychosexual complications.

Drainage

B&L **For further reading see *Bailey and Love*, p.266.**

How are drains used in surgery?

Drainage can be established operatively by channeling the contents of the internal organs externally (ileostomy, colostomy, urostomy, cholecystectomy) or by diverting the visceral contents internally (gastric drainage via pyloroplasty or gastroenterostomy, cholecystojejunostomy or ureterosigmoidostomy).

Drains can be used to remove:

- normal organ contents (e.g. Foley's catheter for urine, nasogastric tube for gastric contents, extraventricular drains for cerebrospinal fluid, and chest drain for pleural fluid)
- abnormal organ contents: pus, blood and air.

What are the indications for inserting drains in surgery?
- Removal of harmful substances (nidus of infection)
- Removal of dead space (e.g. third-space pooling)
- Monitoring and preventing operative complications (e.g. haemorrhage and anastomotic leak)
- Creating a therapeutic tract (e.g. t-tube tract).

What are the types of drain?
Active systems
- *Open:* sump drain (an inner tube under suction is protected from blockage by an outer vented/irrigated tube)
- *Closed:* Redivac drain and chest drain (connected to an underwater seal).

Passive systems
- *Open:* ribbon gauze wick, seton and corrugated drain
- *Closed:* Robinson drain.

What are the potential complications of surgical drains?
- Infection
- Damage to surrounding structures – bowel (anastomotic leakage, perforation, fistula formation); vessels (bleeding); nerves (motor and sensory disruption)
- Obstruction
- Migration
- Displacement.

→ ## Adhesions

For further reading see *Bailey and Love*, Chapter 66.

What is an adhesion?
An adhesion is the union of two normally separate surfaces connected by fibrous connective tissue in an inflamed or damaged region. Adhesions may be classified into various types according to whether they are early (fibrinous) or late (fibrous), or by their underlying aetiology.

What do adhesions cause?
Adhesions are the commonest cause of intestinal obstruction in the West. They account for one-third of all cases of intestinal obstructions in general and 50 per cent of small bowel obstructions. Adhesions can lead to bowel strangulation. They are also responsible for causing chronic pain, and pelvic adhesions can result in infertility.

How may adhesions be classified?

Congenital (2 per cent)
- Meckel's diverticulum
- Malrotation of colon
- Congenital bands.

Acquired (98 per cent)
- Postoperative (80 per cent)
- Postinflammatory (18 per cent)
- Acute appendicitis, diverticulitis, cholecystitis, pelvic infection, and inflammatory bowel disease (Crohn's disease and ulcerative colitis).

How are adhesions managed?

Preoperative
- Conservative treatment – nasogastric suction and intravenous fluids ('drip and suck')
- Nutritional support.

Operative
- Surgical relief – bypass, resection and adhesiolysis
- Preventative measures to avoid further adhesions (practical and theoretical):
  - use of powder-free gloves
  - minimal handling of bowel
  - instillation of various fluids (dextran 70, iodine) or gas into the peritoneal cavity to hold damaged surfaces apart
  - enhancement of peristalsis to disrupt early fibrinous adhesions which have the potential to become fibrous adhesions if left
  - covering anastomosis and raw peritoneal surfaces with inert membranes, lubricants or grafts of peritoneum (e.g. greater omentum placed between the bowel and abdominal wall)
  - use of enzymes to digest adhesions (e.g. trypsin and hyaluronidase)
  - instillation of substances to inhibit deposition of fibrin (fibrinolytic agents, steroids).

Postoperative
- Conservative treatment – nasogastric suction and IV fluids ('drip and suck')
- Nutritional support
- Antibiotics (if clinically indicated)
- Early mobilisation
- Early use of enteral feeding.

What are the causes of sudden death in surgery?

Anaesthetic causes
Hypoxia:
- Respiratory obstruction (including kinked or displaced endotracheal tube)
- Vagal stimulation
- Disconnection from ventilator
- Tension pneumothorax secondary to positive-pressure ventilation
- Mendelson syndrome or chemical pneumonitis (due to hydrochloric acid aspiration during induction)
- Shock (undetected hypotension secondary to internal bleeding)
- Embolisation (venous, air, fat).

Medication:
- Inappropriate drugs administered
- Anaphylactic reaction (drugs or blood)
- Overdose of medication (local anaesthetic)
- Cardiac dysrhythmias (vasodilators, ganglion blocks, diuretics)
- Electrolyte and metabolic imbalances
- Opiates.

Surgical causes
- Hypotension (manipulation of bowel, mesenteric stretching or sympathectomy)
- Cardiac arrhythmia (induced by catheterisation, cardiac surgery)
- Oculocardiac reflex (patient in prone position with direct pressure on eyes causing vagal stimulation)
- Damage to surrounding nerves, arteries and veins (e.g. incision of a groin aneurysm during a hernia repair).

Patient causes
Myocardial infarction, pulmonary oedema, pulmonary embolism, stroke, dehydration, electrolyte imbalances.

Sutures

B&L **For further reading see *Bailey and Love*, Chapter 18.**
The examiner may ask you to demonstrate your surgical skills in suturing. Practise your technique on models and patients prior to the examination.

What is a suture?
A suture is a material used to tie or approximate tissues together. (A suture is also a joint with minimal connective tissue located in the skull vault – e.g. coronal and sagittal sutures.)

What are the types of suture?

Sutures are classified as follows: absorbable versus non-absorbable; natural versus synthetic; and monofilament versus polyfilament (braided). Sutures may also be classified by size (5/0, 4/0, 3/0 etc.).

- *Absorbable:* PDS (polydioxanone); vicryl (polyglactin); monocryl
- *Non-absorbable:* steel; prolene (polypropylene); nylon (ethilon); silk
- *Natural:* silk; catgut
- *Synthetic:* vicryl; PDS
- *Monofilament:* PDS; prolene
- *Polyfilament/braided:* vicryl; silk.

How are sutures broken down?

- Proteolytic digestion (e.g. catgut)
- Hydrolysis (e.g. vicryl).

What makes a good suture material?

An ideal suture:

- is all-purpose (can be used for all types of surgery)
- is easy to handle
- maintains adequate tensile strength
- causes minimal tissue reaction
- holds securely
- has no memory
- is resistant to shrinkage
- is inexpensive
- is easily sterilised
- has predictable performance
- has high breaking strength
- is inert (non-electrolytic, non-capillary, non-allergenic and non-carcinogenic).

What type of suture is vicryl?

Vicryl (polyglactin) is an absorbable, synthetic, braided polymeric suture. It produces a minimal tissue reaction. It is fully absorbed after 56–70 days, and provides adequate support for around 30 days.

What type of suture is silk?

Silk is a non-absorbable, natural, braided suture. It is biodegradable. Its tensile strength lasts up to one year. It causes an inflammatory tissue reaction and should be avoided in the placement of vascular prostheses or artifical heart valves.

Needles

B&L For further reading see *Bailey and Love*, Chapter 18.

What are the parts of a needle?

A needle is compromised of its point, body and swage.

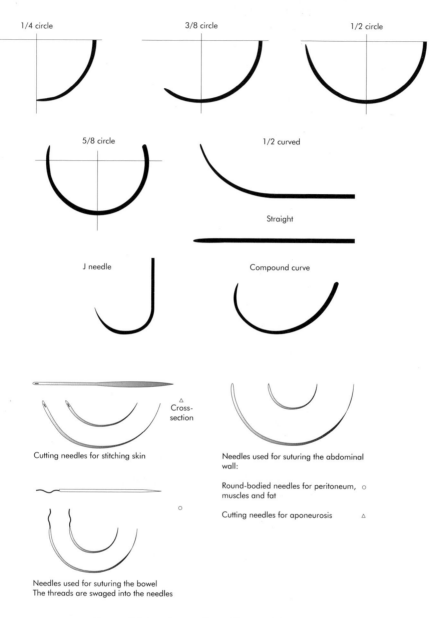

Figure 3.3 ● Types of needles used for sutures. The sutures are swaged on to prevent a 'shoulder' and allow easy passage through tissues. (Bailey and Love, Figure 18.6, p. 241.)

How are needles classified?

Needles can be classified by shape, type and effect (Fig. 3.3).

Shape

■ Straight
■ Curved: 1/4, 3/8, 1/2 and 5/8 circle

■ J-shaped
■ Compound curve.

Type

Round-bodied needles:

These are designed to separate (not cut) tissue fibres. They may be used in soft tissues. After the needle is passed, the tissue closes tightly around the suture material to form a leakproof line. Types are:

■ intestinal
■ heavy
■ blunt taper-point
■ blunt point.

Cutting needles:

These are designed for tough or dense tissues. Types are:

■ tapercut
■ conventional cutting
■ reverse cutting.

Effect

■ *Traumatic needles* are with holes or eyes. They are supplied separate from the suture thread. The suture is threaded on-site. A needle with an eye carries ? double strand, which creates a larger hole and disruption to the underlying tissue. These are rarely seen nowadays but are occasionally still used (e.g. aneurysm needle).
■ *Atraumatic needles* are eyeless and are swaged (pre-mounted) to a suture. This reduces handling and preparation time and causes less trauma to the underlying tissues.

What advantage does a reverse cutting needle have over a cutting needle?

In a reverse cutting needle the cutting edge is situated on the outside of the needle and is therefore less likely to cut through the tissues. In addition, by having the apex cutting edge on the outside of the needle curvature, this improves the strength of the needle and increases its resistance to bending.

How are surgical needles chosen?

Remember the mnemonic PATS:

■ **P** = **p**rocedure
■ **A** = **a**ccess
■ **T** = **t**issue
■ **S** = **s**urgeon's preference.

$B\&L$ For further reading see *Bailey and Love*, Chapter 17.

What is the normal daily resting energy expenditure of a 70 kg man?

He uses 1800 kcal.

What are the daily protein/nitrogen requirements for healthy and critically ill patients?

- Healthy patient requires 0.15 g/kg of nitrogen
- Critically ill patient requires 0.3 g/kg of nitrogen.

What routes of nutrition are available, and why are they chosen?

See Fig. 3.4.

- *Enteral* nutrition is used in patients with a normally functioning gastrointestinal tract. Feeding routes are oral, nasogastric, nasojejunal, nasoduodenal and tube enterostomy.
- *Parenteral* nutrition is the treatment of choice in patients with catabolic states and non-functioning gastrointestinal tracts.

If enteral feeding is preferred, what are the indications for total parenteral nutrition?

- Patient who cannot ingest food

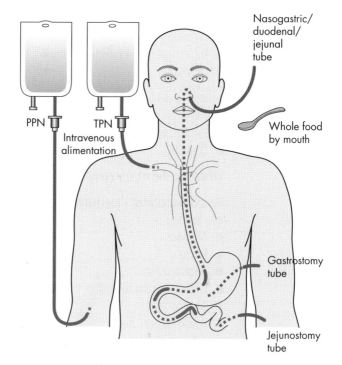

Figure 3.4 ● Techniques used for adjuvant nutritional support. PPN, partial parenteral nutrition; TPN, total parenteral nutrition. Redrawn with permission from Nick Tharp, rxkinetics.com. (Bailey and Love, Figure 17.5, p.229.)

Nasogastric/ duodenal/ jejunal tube

PPN

TPN
Intravenous alimentation

Whole food by mouth

Gastrostomy tube

Jejunostomy tube

- Anorexia:
  - neurological disorders
  - posterior fossa cranial surgery
  - head injury
  - coma (reduced GCS)
- Trauma and tumours (involving the maxilla, head or neck):
  - patients with malfunctioning gastrointestinal tract
  - short-bowel syndrome secondary to small bowel resection
  - fistula (enteroenteric, enterocolic, enterovesical, enterocutaneous)
  - obstruction (GI tumours, strictures, adhesions, pyloric obstruction)
  - paralytic ileus
  - inflammatory disease (Crohn's disease, ulcerative colitis, pancreatitis diverticular disease, radiation enteritis)
  - peptic ulceration
  - mesenteric vascular occlusion (ischaemia)
  - malignancy
  - trauma
- Hypercatabolic states
- Major GI anomalies (tracheo-oesphageal fistula, gastroschisis, and intestinal atresia).

What are the major complications of enteral feeding?

Related to intubation of GI tract

- Fistulation
- Wound infection
- Peritonitis
- Displacement and catheter migration
- Obstruction of the tube.

Related to delivery of nutrient to GI tract

- Aspiration or pneumonia
- Feed intolerance
- Diarrhoea.

What are the major complications of parenteral feeding?

Related to catheter – mechanical

- Blockage
- Migration
- Fracture
- Displacement
- Central vein thrombosis
- Air embolism
- Pneumothorax, haemothorax or hydrothorax
- Subclavian artery and vein injury
- Cardiac arrhythmias (if catheter is placed in the ventricle).

Related to catheter – infective

- Exit site skin infection
- Line sepsis
- Infective endocarditis.

Metabolic

- Hyper- or hypoglycaemia
- Hypertriglyceridaemia
- Hyperchloraemic acidosis
- Hypo-kalaemia, -magnesaemia and -phosphataemia
- Essential fatty acid deficiency
- Deranged liver function tests.

Metabolic response to surgery

B&L **For further reading see *Bailey and Love*, Chapter 1.**

What is the metabolic response to surgery?

The metabolic response to surgery is described by the 'ebb and flow' model (Fig. 3.5).

The ebb phase

This phase begins at the time of surgery (injury) and is characterised by hypovolaemia, depression of metabolic rate, reduced cardiac output, hypothermia, lactic acidosis and an overall reduction in energy expenditure. The main hormones in this phase are catecholamines, cortisol and aldosterone.

The flow phase

This phase is divided into the catabolic and anabolic phases.

- In the catabolic phase, there is an increased catecholamine drive and energy is mobilised from adipose tissue and carbohydrate stores in the liver and muscle to aid recovery and repair. This phase is characterised by tissue oedema, increased metabolic rate, increased cardiac output, increased oxygen consumption and increased gluconeogenesis. Moreover, there is an increased production of hormones (catecholamines, cortisol, insulin, glucagons) and inflammatory cytokines (IL-1, IL-6, TNFα) that utilises fat and protein stores. This leads to weight and nitrogen loss. The increased production of insulin results in insulin resistance. During this phase, the patient is at risk of infections and cardiac dysfunction.
- The anabolic phase occurs in conjunction with repair. There is weight gain, and protein and fat stores increase, and the metabolic response returns to normal.

How long does each metabolic phase last?

The ebb phase lasts 24–48 hours. The catabolic flow phase lasts between 3 and 10 days. The anabolic flow phase lasts from weeks to months.

- Alpha-fetoprotein screening is used to detect certain fetal abnormalities in pregnant women.
- Cancer screening is an attempt to prevent cancer, or diagnose it in its early stages. For example, the Pap smear is used to detect potentially precancerous lesions and prevent cervical cancer.

Name a current screening programme available in England.
In 1988, The National Health Service Breast Screening Programme was introduced. It provides free breast screening (mammography) every three years for all women over 50 years of age.

Audit and clinical governance

B&L   **For further reading see *Bailey and Love*, Chapter 8.**

What is an audit?
It is a systematic process by which a group of professionals review a current system of practice, to identify weakness, make changes and monitor the standard of practice.

According to the National Institute for Clinical Excellence (NICE), it is 'a quality improvement process that seeks to improve patient care and outcome through systematic review of care against explicit criteria and the implementation of change'.

Outline some types of audit.
- Standards-based audit is a cycle that involves defining standards, collecting data to measure current practice against those standards, and implementing any changes deemed necessary.
- Peer review is an assessment of the quality of care provided by a clinical team with a view to improving clinical care. Peers discuss individual cases.
- Adverse occurrence screening and critical incident monitoring is used to peer review cases that had adverse or unexpected outcomes. A multidisciplinary team discusses individual cases, addresses the way the team functioned and what can be learnt for the future.
- Patient surveys and focus groups allow patients' views about the quality of care to be heard.

What is the audit cycle?
The clinical audit cycle is a systematic process of establishing best practice; measuring against criteria, taking action to improve care and monitoring to achieve improvement.
- Stage 1: Identify the problem.
- Stage 2: Define criteria and standards.
- Stage 3: Data collection.
- Stage 4: Compare performance with criteria and standards.
- Stage 5: Implement change.
- Stage 6: Re-audit – close the audit loop.

What is clinical governance?

Clinical governance is the term used to describe a systematic approach of maintaining and improving the quality of patient care within a healthcare system. According to Scally and Donaldson (1998), it is 'a framework through which NHS organisations are accountable for continually improving the quality of their services and safeguarding high standards of care by creating an environment in which excellence in clinical care will flourish'. There are three key attributes:

- maintaining high standards of care
- transparent responsibility and accountability for standards
- aiming for constant improvement.

What are the 'seven pillars of clinical governance'?

- Audit
- Education and training: continuing professional development
- Clinical effectiveness and research (evidence-based medicine)
- Risk management
- Patient and public involvement
- Information technology
- Staff management.

Research and statistics

B&L **For further reading see *Bailey and Love*, Chapter 8.**

What is a controlled clinical trial?

A controlled trial is a scientific experiment in which one or more treatments are compared with a control treatment. The controls may be non-treatment, placebo or a standard clinical practice.

What is a crossover design for clinical trials?

In crossover designs, the patient acts as his or her own control. Treatments are compared and their order is randomised.

What is randomisation?

Randomisation is a method of assigning subjects to an experimental or control arm of a study. Each patient has an equal chance of appearing in either treatment group. It helps avoid selection bias.

What is meant by blinding?

Blinding is a method used to eliminate any bias inherent in the data collection. A study is single-blinded if the patient is unaware of the treatment allocation. In the best randomised controlled trials, neither patient nor researcher is aware of which therapy has been used until after the study has been conducted (double-blinded).

What are type I and type II errors?

- Type I errors occur when the null hypothesis (HO) is rejected when it is in fact true. In other words, benefit is perceived when really there is none (false positive).

■ Type II errors occur when the null hypothesis (HO) is not rejected when it is in fact false. In other words, benefit is missed when it was there to be found (false negative).

What is the power of a trial?

The power measures the sensitivity of the trial to detect a difference and is equal to a type II error.

What does it mean to state that a result is 'statistically significant'?

The result is unlikely to have occurred by chance. Normally this equates to a p-value of less than 0.05 (5 per cent).

What is a 'confidence interval' (CI)?

It is an interval estimate of any population parameter. It is used to indicate the reliability of an estimate. The CI provides the probability that a true population is contained within a range from a sample mean and its standard error.

Fractures

B&L **For further reading see** *Bailey and Love*, **Chapter 27.**

What is a fracture?

A fracture is a break in the continuity of a bone. It may be complete or incomplete (based on whether both cortices are involved), or open or closed (based on whether the overlying skin is intact).

What are the phases of bone healing?

■ *Reactive phase*: fracture and inflammation, followed by granulation tissue formation
■ *Reparative phase*: callus formation and lamellar bone deposition
■ *Remodelling phase*: remodelling to the original bone contour.

What classification do you know for proximal femoral fractures?

The Garden classification:
■ I: incomplete fractures (including impacted valgus fracture)
■ II: complete fracture without displacement
■ III: complete fracture with partial displacement
■ IV: complete fracture with full displacement.

How may fractures be treated?

The treatment of bone fractures depends on the type and location of the fracture and the patient's age and medical history. However, four phases can be identified (the 4 Rs):
■ Resuscitation
■ Reduction (open or closed)
■ Restriction (immobilisation) (cast splint, functional brace, continuous traction, internal fixation, external fixation)
■ Rehabilitation (physiotherapy).

What are the early complications of fractures?

Local

- Vascular injury causing haemorrhaging (internal or external)
- Visceral injury causing damage to the surrounding organs (e.g. brain, lung or bladder)
- Damage to surrounding soft tissue, nerves or skin
- Haemarthrosis
- Compartment syndrome (or Volkmann's ischaemia)
- Wound infection.

Systemic

- Fat embolism
- Shock
- Thromboembolism (pulmonary or venous)
- Exacerbation of underlying diseases (diabetes, ischaemic heart disease)
- Pneumonia.

What are the late complications of fractures?

Local

- Delayed union
- Non-union
- Mal-union
- Joint stiffness
- Contractures
- Infection
- Myositis ossificans
- Avascular necrosis
- Algodystrophy (Sudeck's atrophy)
- Osteomyelitis
- Growth disturbance or deformity.

Systemic

- Gangrene, tetanus, septicaemia
- Fear of mobilising (compensation neurosis)
- Osteoarthritis.

Sterilisation

B&L For further reading see *Bailey and Love*, Chapter 15.

What is meant by cleaning?

Cleaning is the process of physical removal of organic debris (e.g. blood, tissue and other body fluids) but does not necessarily destroy micro-organisms.

What is disinfection?
Disinfection reduces the number of viable organisms.

What is sterilisation?
Sterilisation refers to the process that kills or eliminates transmissible viable micro-organisms (bacteria, viruses, fungi, spores, cysts).

How may the methods of sterilisation be classified?

Physical sterilisation
- Heat sterilisation with moist heat (pressurised steam autoclaves) at 134°C
- Heat sterilisation with dry heat at 160°C
- Radiation sterilisation.

Chemical sterilisation
- Ethylene oxide
- Ozone
- Chlorine bleach
- Formaldehyde
- Glutaraldehyde
- Hydrogen peroxide
- Peracetic acid
- Ethanol (70 per cent).

Give some examples of sterilisation.
- Moist heat sterilisation (steam autoclaves) for trays of surgical instruments
- Dry heat sterilisation for non-aqueous liquids and ointments
- Ionising radiation for swabs, catheters and syringes
- Ethylene oxide for sutures and electrical equipment
- Formaldehyde for plastics
- Glutaraldehyde for endoscopes.

Does sterilisation destroy prions?
No.

Prior to sterilisation of your surgical instruments, what do you need to do?
All instruments need to be cleaned and thoroughly dried before they are sterilised. There are three main cleaning methods: hand scrubbing, ultrasonic cleaning and automated washing.

What types of disinfectants do you use when scrubbing?
See Fig. 3.6.

Chlorhexidine gluconate is an aqueous quaternary ammonium compound. It has a residual effect and is effective for more than 4 hours. It has potent antiseptic activity against Gram-positive and Gram-negative organisms and some viruses, but only moderate activity against the tubercle bacillus. It has poor activity against spores and fungi.

Povidone-iodine is a potent bactericidal, fungicidal and viricidal agent. There is some activity against bacterial spores and good activity against tubercle bacillus. The iodine penetrates cell walls to produce antimicrobial effects. Iodine has some residual effects but these are not sustained for more than 4 hours. In addition, it may cause irritation to the skin or allergic reactions.

Alcohols are rapid-acting antimicrobial agents with broad-spectrum activity. They are effective in destroying Gram-positive and Gram-negative bacteria, fungi, viruses and tubercle bacillus. However, they are not sporicidal.

Antibacterial prophylaxis

B&L **Please refer to *Bailey and Love*, Chapter 4.**

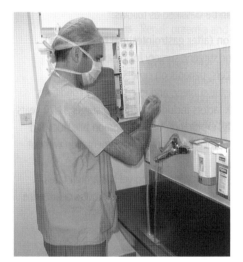

What is an antibiotic?

An antibiotic is a substance, produced by or derived from a micro-organism, that destroys or inhibits the growth of other micro-organisms.

How may wound contamination be classified?

See Table 3.1.

(a)

Figure 3.6 ●
Scrubbing up.
(*Bailey and Love*,
Figures 15.4a,
p.208 and 15.4b,
p.208.)

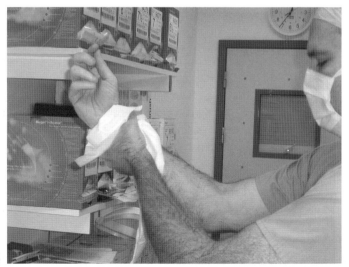

(b)

- A patient should not fast for prolonged periods, but be scheduled **first** on an operating list.
- *Diet-controlled diabetic patients:*
  - For minor surgery, no additional precautions are required.
  - For major surgery, monitor blood glucose and if elevated commence an insulin sliding scale.
- *Oral hypoglycaemic-controlled diabetic patients:*
  - For minor surgery, the morning dose of the oral hypoglycaemic agent should be omitted. It is restarted once the patient is eating and drinking. Continue to monitor blood glucose levels.
  - For major surgery, the patient should be commenced on an insulin sliding scale when they are nil by mouth and stopped when they have resumed eating and drinking.
- *Insulin-controlled diabetic patients:*
  - For all surgeries, the insulin dose should not be given while the patient is fasted. They should be commenced on an insulin sliding scale with dextrose infusion. This may be stopped when the patient has resumed eating and drinking.

Intraoperative period

- Anaesthesia combined with surgical stress has a definite hyperglycaemic effect.
- Consider local, regional, spinal or epidural anaesthesia. Moreover, a general anaesthetic is tolerated in most diabetics.
- Blood pressure and blood glucose should be monitored throughout surgery.

Postoperative period

- Aim to have the patient's blood glucose levels within normal range.
- Oral fluids once started should be followed by a soft diet and then a diabetic diet. Normal regimes may then be resumed.
- Monitor for symptoms and signs of infection.

HIV in surgery

B&L **For further reading see *Bailey and Love*, Chapter 4.**

What is HIV?

Human immunodeficiency virus (HIV) is a lentivirus (a member of the retrovirus family) that may lead to acquired immunodeficiency syndrome (AIDS). In 1981, AIDS was first identified in Los Angeles. The virus destroys helper (CD4) T-cells resulting in the suppression of the body's immune response.

Who is at high risk of acquiring the infection?

- *Sexual activity*: unprotected sexual relations, including homosexual males

- *Blood products*: intravenous drug use; haemophiliacs (before 1985) and recipients of blood and blood products
- *Mother to child*: *in utero*; intrapartum; and breast-feeding
- *Endemic areas*: Africa and South East Asia.

How long does it take to seroconvert?

In 85 per cent of cases, seroconversion occurs within 12 weeks of infection.

How are doctors and other health workers at risk?

While treating patients, we are commonly exposed to bodily fluids (including blood). This can occur with needlestick injuries, mucosal contact and bodily fluid spillages and splashes.

What is the risk of HIV transmission following exposure with infected blood?

See Table 3.2.

Table 3.2
HIV risk following exposure to an infected source

Route	Estimated infections/ 10 000 exposures	Percentage
Blood transfusion	9000	90%
Needle sharing	67	0.67%
Percutaneous needlestick	30	0.3%

What factors increase the risk of seroconversion following needlestick injuries?

- Exposure to large inoculation of blood
- Deep penetrating injury
- Visible blood on the needle
- Procedures that cannulate blood vessels (arterial blood gases, central lines)
- Patient with high viral loads and low CD4 counts
- HIV progression (AIDS).

When should you consider administering post-exposure prophylaxis (PEP)?

The uptake and processing of the HIV antigen may take several hours to days. There is a window of opportunity for prevention. In the UK, prophylaxis is recommended for high-risk individuals. A set protocol should be followed.

Immediate action

Following any exposure the site is washed liberally with soap and water (without scrubbing). Free bleeding of puncture wounds should be encouraged. Exposed mucous membranes, including conjunctivae, should be irrigated copiously with water, before and after removing any contact lenses.

Risk assessment

This assessment needs to be made urgently by someone other than the exposed worker about the appropriateness of starting treatment. Consideration should also be given to risk of exposure to hepatitis B and C. The decision for prophylaxis is based on the exposure potential, the type of body fluid or substance involved, and the route and severity of exposure. There are three types of exposure in healthcare settings associated with significant risk:

- percutaneous injury from needles, instruments, bone fragments, and significant bites that break the skin
- exposure of broken skin (abrasions, cuts, eczema)
- exposure of mucous membranes, including the eye.

Prescribing PEP

PEP should be recommended to healthcare workers if they have had a significant occupational exposure to blood, or high-risk body fluid from a patient, or other source, either known to be HIV infected, or considered to be at high risk of HIV infection. PEP is generally not offered after exposure through any route with low-risk materials (urine, vomit, saliva, faeces) unless they are visibly blood-stained. It is important to take into account the views of the exposed healthcare worker.

What is the recommended medication for PEP?

The recommended medications in PEP starter packs include:

- zidovudine 250 mg or 300 mg b.d.
- lamivudine 150 mg b.d.
- nelfinavir 1250 mg b.d. or 750 mg t.d.s.

Critical care

Introduction

Critical care is examined by direct viva and through written questions. An understanding of basic physiological principles is essential to competently answer the probing management-style questions.

Airways and ventilation

B&L For further reading see *Bailey and Love*, Chapter 14.

How would you assess a patient's airway?

- *Look*: symmetrical chest wall movement; use of accessory muscles; foreign body in the airway; 'see-saw' breathing
- *Listen*: coughing; gagging; choking; stridor; gurgling
- *Feel*: chest wall movements; oronasal air flow.

What options do you have to manage the airway?

- *Manoeuvres*: suction; head tilt; chin lift; jaw thrust
- *Adjuncts*: oro/naso-pharyngeal airways
- *Definitive*: oro/naso-tracheal intubation; surgical airway (cricothyroidotomy, tracheostomy).

List the types of tracheostomy.

- Elective versus emergency
- Cuffed versus uncuffed
- Fenestrated versus unfenestrated
- Open versus percutaneous
- Silver metal versus plastic.

What complications are associated with a tracheostomy?

- Bleeding – may aspirate
- Subcutaneous emphysema
- Local infection
- Tracheal stenosis
- Damage to brachiocephalic vein from misplacement with tube change.

How might ventilation be assisted?

- Non-invasive positive-pressure ventilation (e.g. BIPAP, CPAP)
- Invasive positive-pressure ventilation.

Which conditions may benefit from non-invasive positive-pressure ventilation?

- Exacerbation of chronic obstructive pulmonary disease (COPD)
- Acute pulmonary oedema
- Pneumonia
- Facilitation of weaning from mechanical (invasive) ventilation.

What are the types of mechanical ventilators, and how do they work?

- *Types*: volume-cycled (delivers preset volume); pressure-cycled (delivers preset pressure); flow-cycled (delivers preset flow); time-cycled (delivers preset frequency)
- *Modes*: controlled mechanical or continuous mandatory (ventilates regardless of inspiratory effort); assist-controlled (ventilates in response to inspiratory effort and if absent effort); synchronous intermittent (ventilates supplementary to spontaneous breathing)
- *Adjuncts*: positive end-expiratory pressure (PEEP); continuous positive airway pressure (CPAP).

Acid–base

Can you interpret this arterial blood gas profile?

See Fig. 4.1.

What could be causing it?

Respiratory causes

- *Acidosis*: hypoventilation which has both central causes (depression of the respiratory centres, e.g. by opioids, GAs) and peripheral causes (acute respiratory failure (type II), airway obstruction and decreased chest wall movement, e.g. trauma)
- *Alkalosis*: hyperventilation (e.g. fever, sepsis, pain, anxiety, pneumonia, pulmonary embolus).

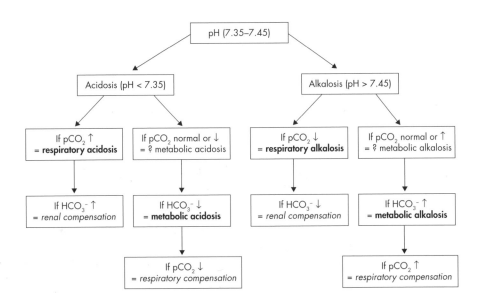

Figure 4.1 ● Arterial blood gas profile.

Metabolic causes
■ *Acidosis* with raised anion gap:
- raised lactic acid (secondary to shock, infection and hypoxia)
- raised ketoacids (secondary to diabetes mellitus, alcohol)
- 'fixed' acids (renal failure)
- ingested acids (drugs and toxins)

■ *Acidosis* with normal anion gap (e.g. diarrhoea, fistulae, renal tubular acidosis)

■ *Alkalosis*: excess loss of acid (e.g. vomiting).

What are the commonest causes of new-onset dyspnoea several days after an operation?
■ Pulmonary embolus
■ Pneumonia
■ Myocardial infarction and pulmonary oedema
■ Bronchospasm
■ Pneumothorax.

How would you investigate and treat new-onset dyspnoea?
■ History and physical examination
■ Arterial blood gasses (ABG)
■ Blood profile: haematology (? raised white cell count); CRP; coagulation (D-dimer)
■ Chest X-ray
■ Electrocardiogram
■ Ventilation/perfusion (V/Q) scan; CT pulmonary angiogram
■ Deep-vein Doppler study
■ Antibiotic therapy for pneumonia
■ Anticoagulation for pulmonary embolus.

→ ## Case study

You are having a busy weekend on call and your FY1 (Foundation Year 1) has just returned from seeing a patient with a history of alcoholic liver disease and atrial fibrillation, now presenting with non-specific abdominal pain. Your FY1 hands you the patient's arterial blood gas profile while telling you the patient is a poor historian and is being disruptive in A&E. The arterial blood gases show the following: pH=7.32; PCO_2=3.43 kPa; PO_2=14.4 kPa; HCO_3^-=17 mmol/L. Your FY1 has almost lost his patience with this patient and feels that the patient is just intoxicated.

Do you agree? What would you do next?
The patient may well be intoxicated, but he has a metabolic acidosis with respiratory compensation. In view of the clinical history, and symptoms and signs, bowel ischaemia secondary to a mesenteric embolic event must be excluded. This is potentially a surgical emergency. The patient urgently needs resuscitation, a more senior surgical review, followed by CT imaging and laparotomy.

What else could you calculate? What else would you ask for?
You could calculate the anion gap which you would expect to be raised. A lactate level would also be helpful.

Burns

B&L **For further reading see *Bailey and Love*, Chapter 28.**

How would you assess a patient presenting with a burn injury?
- A – B – C – D – E
- Careful assessment for inhalational injury (facial burns, singed hair, cough, sooty sputum) with a low threshold for intubation
- Wallace's 'rule of nines' (percentages): head=9; single arm=9; anterior trunk=18; posterior trunk=18; single leg=18; genitalia=1
- Thickness: partial-thickness (red/white, blistering, sensate) versus full-thickness (white, leathery, desensate)
- Early discussion with burns unit to arrange transfer if necessary.

How would you resuscitate a patient presenting with a burn injury?
In addition to maintenance fluid, replacement crystalloids are given at 4 mL/kg for each percentage burn of total body surface area, over 24 hours (Parkland formula). Fifty per cent of the total calculated volume is given in the first 8 hours.

What complications should you be vigilant for?
- Shock from fluid and electrolyte losses
- Sepsis
- Acute respiratory distress syndrome (ARDS)
- Constricting effect of circumferential burns – may cause ischaemia (e.g. if on the limbs) or ventilatory problems (e.g. if chest wall burns) which may require escharotomy
- Renal failure secondary to myoglobinuria.

Intensive care unit (ICU)

B&L **For further reading see *Bailey and Love*, Chapter 16.**

Which patients are appropriate to be referred to the ICU?
- Those needing advanced respiratory support
- Those needing mechanical support of two or more organ systems
- Those needing close and/or invasive monitoring of organ dysfunction
- Those needing intensive nursing input (usually one to one)
- Those in whom the condition is potentially reversible.

What is shock? How is it classified and graded?
Shock is inadequate tissue perfusion secondary to acute circulatory failure. It can be hypovolaemic, septic, anaphylactic, cardiogenic or neurogenic. There are four grades of severity:

- Grade 1 (0–15 per cent, 0–750 mL): tachycardia
- Grade 2 (15–30 per cent, 750–1500 mL): tachycardia, narrow pulse pressure, tachypnoea, anxiety
- Grade 3 (30–40 per cent, 1500–2000 mL): tachycardia, tachypnoea, confusion, reduced urine output, reduced systolic BP
- Grade 4 (>40 per cent, >2000 mL): tachycardia, coma, low urine output, unrecordable diastolic BP.

What is the systemic inflammatory response syndrome (SIRS)? What can cause it?

SIRS is a systemic response to the inflammation of endothelium. It is defined by two or more of the following:

- Temperature < 36°C or > 38°C
- Heart rate > 90/min
- Respiratory rate > 20/min or $PaCO_2$ < 4.3 kPa
- White cell count > 12×10^9/L or < 4×10^9/L.

Causes include:

- **i**njury (e.g. burns, trauma)
- **i**nflammation (e.g. acute pancreatitis)
- **i**nfection (e.g. aspiration, faecal peritonitis)
- **i**schaemia (e.g. shock of any cause, reperfusion injury)
- **i**atrogenic (e.g. major surgery, blood transfusions)
- **i**ntoxication
- **i**mmunologic
- **i**diopathic.

How should a neutropenic patient be managed?

- A – B – C – D – E
- History: malignancy, recent chemotherapy, immunosuppressants, HIV, recent transfusion
- Physical examination: signs of sepsis (fever, shock), peripheral/central vascular lines, systems review
- Septic screen: chest X-ray, blood haematology and biochemistry, cultures (blood, sputum, urine, stool, wound swabs, CSF)
- Broad-spectrum antibiotics in accordance with local guidelines and microbiologist advice
- Investigate source of infection: further imaging (e.g. CT, bronchoscopy).

Pancreatitis

B&L **For further reading see *Bailey and Love*, pp.1139–1146.**

How should a patient presenting with pancreatitis be managed?

- A – B – C – D – E and fluid resuscitation
- History: establish cause (gallstones, alcohol, trauma, steroids, mumps,

autoimmunity, hyperlipidaemia, hypercalcaemia, ERCP, drugs, scorpion venom)
- Physical examination
- Arterial blood gases: assess pH and PO_2
- Blood profile: full blood count, liver function, electrolytes, urea, albumin, glucose
- Ultrasound scan: to check for gallstones (may require urgent ERCP and sphincterotomy).

Assess prognostic severity with (e.g.) the modified Glasgow (Imrie) scoring: 1 point for each criterion met on admission and again at 48 hours after admission (1–2 points is associated with a mortality of <1 per cent, 3–4 points with 15 per cent, and 6 points with a mortality approaching 100 per cent) (Table 4.1).

Table 4.1
Modified Glasgow (Imrie) scoring

PO$_2$	< 8 kPa (60 mmHg)
Age	> 55
Neutr/WCC	> 15 × 10^9/L
Ca (corrected)	< 2 mmol/L
Raised Ur	> 16 mmol/L
Enzymes (LDH)	> 600 IU/L
Albumin	< 32 g/L
Sugar (glucose)	> 10 mmol/L

CT performed at 5–7 days after admission can demonstrate features of pancreatitis ranging from mild to severe; i.e. oedema, extrapancreatic changes, fluid collection, necrosis.

What complications may arise from pancreatitis?
- Death (approximately 10 per cent)
- *Local complications*: phlegmon, pseudocyst, abscess, ascites, haemorrhage, necrotising pancreatitis, splenic vein thrombosis, fat necrosis
- *Intestinal complications*: paralytic ileus, gastrointestinal haemorrhage
- *Hepatobiliary complications*: jaundice, stricture of the common bile duct, portal vein thrombosis
- *Systemic complications*:
  - metabolic (malnutrition, hypocalcaemia, hyperglycaemia, hypoalbuminaemia)
  - haematological (disseminated intravascular coagulation)
  - renal (acute renal failure)
  - cardiovascular (circulatory failure (shock), arrhythmias)
  - respiratory (hypoxic acute respiratory failure (ARDS), pleural effusions).

Renal failure

_B&L_ For further reading see _Bailey and Love_, Chapter 20.

What are the causes of acute renal failure following surgery?

- _Prerenal causes_: hypotension, hypovolaemia
- _Renal causes_: nephrotoxic drugs (NSAIDs, gentamicin, ACE inhibitors), sepsis, myoglobinuria, contrast media
- _Postrenal causes_: blocked urinary catheter, ureteric injury, calculi, prostatic obstruction.

What is the commonest cause of renal failure in surgical patients, and why?

The commonest cause is prerenal failure, owing to inadequate renal perfusion secondary to volume depletion.

Where are the commonest surgical fluid losses?

- Haemorrhage
- Gastrointestinal
- Sepsis
- Third space.

What is oliguria, and how should it be managed?

Oliguria is a urine output < 0.5 mL/kg per hour.

- Flush or change the urinary catheter.
- Increase intravenous fluid filling if the patient appears fluid-depleted, but consider cardiac status.
- Institute more invasive monitoring, such as central venous pressure (CVP line) and 'fluid challenge'.
- Consider diuretics (but this may mask the underlying cause).
- Check blood biochemistry: electrolytes and urea (e.g. hyperkalaemia, which may need treating).
- Stop nephrotoxic drugs.
- Treat sepsis aggressively.
- Consider an abdominal ultrasound scan to exclude hydronephrosis from obstructive uropathy.

If there is worsening renal function, increasing fluid retention and electrolyte disturbances, consider dialysis and discuss with the ICU.

Analgesia

_B&L_ For further reading see _Bailey and Love_, Chapter 14.

How should pain relief be prescribed?

Use the WHO 'analgesic ladder': simple analgesics (paracetamol, NSAIDs) > weak opiates (codeine, tramadol, co-codamol) > strong opiates (morphine). Pethidine has been withdrawn from the latest edition of the WHO's guide.

What if the pain is not controlled?

Re-assess the patient for worsening or new pathology. If inadequate analgesia, use an additive approach according to the WHO analgesic ladder (see above). If the pain is still not controlled, discuss with the pain team or anaesthetist for adjuncts and alternatives.

How may analgesics be given?

Enteral:

- Oral (or via nasogastric tube, percutaneous endoscopic gastrostomy etc.)
- Rectal.

Parenteral:

- Intramuscular
- Intravenous
- Subcutaneous (often used in palliative care, e.g. syringe drivers)
- Transdermal (e.g. fentanyl patches)
- Epidural
- Intrathecal
- Local anaesthetic field block.

What is patient-controlled analgesia?

The patient presses a button that delivers a prescribed dose of intravenous or epidural analgesia, at preset intervals, from an electronically controlled infusion pump.

What are the benefits of patient-controlled analgesia?

- Faster pain-sensation to pain-relief time, and thus better pain control
- Objective measure obtained of how much analgesia is required over time
- Reduced nursing input and medication errors.
- There is an internal safety mechanism to prevent opioid overdose because of the 'lockout' time period. If the patient administers too much they fall asleep and stop pressing the button!

Preoperative assessment

B&L   **For further reading see *Bailey and Love*, Chapter 13.**

How should a patient's fitness for surgery be assessed?

- History: previous surgery/anaesthetic, ICU admission, exercise tolerance, medication, smoker, respiratory symptoms
- Physical examination: cardiorespiratory signs (wheeze, cough, dyspnoea, heart murmur, dysrhythmia)
- Electrocardiogram and chest X-ray
- Blood profile: haematology (anaemia, infection), coagulation, biochemistry (renal function)

- Additional investigations:
  - arterial blood gasses
  - lung spirometry (PEFR, FEV_1, FVC)
  - echocardiogram
  - exercise tolerance test.

You should be aware that NICE has produced guidelines on what preoperative investigations are required for individual groups of patients. Recommendations are based on the age of the patient, the ASA grade of patient and the type of surgery.

What should you do if you are concerned about a patient's fitness for surgery?

- Have an early discussion with the anaesthetist performing the list.
- Arrange appropriate specialist consultations early with respect to the areas of concern, specifically asking for approval for surgery.
- If necessary delay the surgical procedure until it is safe to proceed, unless it is an emergency and the risk is outweighed by the gain.
- Inform the operating team and bookings office early regarding possible delays to the surgical procedure.

Jaundice

B&L **For further reading see *Bailey and Love*, Chapter 13.**

What specific questions would you ask a jaundiced patient, and why?

- Presence of pain: painless jaundice may suggest malignancy
- Presence of pale stools and/or dark urine, pruritus: suggests obstruction of the biliary tree (e.g. gallstone, tumour)
- Unintentional weight-loss: suggests a possible malignancy obstructing the biliary tree (e.g. head of pancreas carcinoma, cholangiocarcinoma)
- Foreign travel and/or ingested shellfish: suggests viral hepatitis A
- Recent transfusion: suggests haemolytic anaemia or infective hepatitis
- Family history of jaundice: hereditary conditions (e.g. Crigler–Najjar syndrome)
- Current medications: hepatotoxic drugs
- Alcohol intake: alcoholic hepatitis; cirrhosis
- Intravenous drug abuse and sexual history: infective hepatitis.

What are the causes of jaundice?

Prehepatic causes

- Haemolysis
- Gilbert's syndrome and other congenital enzymatic defects in bilirubin metabolism (e.g. Crigler–Najjar syndrome)
- Dyserythropoiesis.

Hepatocellular causes (cirrhosis)

- Congenital/genetic: haemochromatosis; Wilson's, α_1-antitrypsin deficiency
- Alcohol
- Drugs and toxins
- Autoimmune (e.g. primary biliary cirrhosis)
- Infections: viral hepatitis; leptospirosis; CMV, HIV, EBV etc.
- Neoplasia: primary (hepatocellular carcinoma) and secondary/metastatic
- Cardiac cirrhosis: congestive cardiac failure.

Posthepatic (obstructive) jaundice

- Gallstones within the common bile duct
- Carcinoma of the head of pancreas
- Ascending cholangitis
- Carcinoma around the ampulla of Vater
- Lymphadenopathy at the porta hepatis
- Primary sclerosing cholangitis
- Mirizzi's syndrome
- Benign strictures of the common bile duct:
  - inflammatory (pancreatitis)
  - postoperative
  - after radiotherapy
- Malignant strictures of the common bile duct (cholangiocarcinoma)
- Congenital: biliary atresia.

If you suspect a patient has obstructive jaundice, how would you proceed, and why?

- A – B – C – D – E
- History: as above
- Physical examination: pyrexia; tenderness in right upper quadrant; palpable mass or nodes; palpable gallbladder (Courvoisier's law); urine dipstick; stool sample
- Blood profile: haematology (anaemia, inflammation – cholecystitis/cholangitis); biochemistry (hydration status, hepatorenal syndrome); liver function (ALT, AST, Alk phos, bilirubin, albumin – hepatitic/obstructive picture); coagulation (derangement secondary to liver dysfunction needs correction prior to intervention)
- Blood cultures: if cholangitis suspected
- Ultrasound scan: cholecystitis/cholangitis; gallstones; dilated common bile duct; head of pancreas tumour; cholangiocarcinoma; hepatitis.

How would subsequent management differ following an ultrasound report of an obstructing gallstone from a report of an obstructing tumour mass?

- *Gallstones*: Consider urgent ERCP and sphincterotomy to remove the obstructing gallstone.
- *Tumour*: Requires urgent CT staging and multidisciplinary discussion for subsequent therapy. However, in worsening obstructive jaundice, immediate biliary drainage and stenting may be required initially. This can be performed percutaneously under radiological guidance.

What are the complications of surgery in the jaundiced patient?

- Altered fluid balance: hypoalbuminaemia (leading to peripheral oedema and ascites); secondary hyperaldosteronism (leading to sodium retention and hypokalaemia)
- Acid–base disturbances
- Coagulopathy
- Hepatorenal syndrome (leading to renal failure)
- Altered drug metabolism
- Metabolic derangements (e.g. hypoglycaemia)
- Increased risk of sepsis
- Delayed wound healing
- Malnutrition
- Hepatic encephalopathy
- Increased risk to hospital staff (if infective hepatitis).

Trauma

B&L **For further reading see *Bailey and Love*, Chapter 22.**

How would you manage a patient brought in from a road traffic accident who is tachycardic?

- A + cervical spine control – B – C – D – E
- Fluid resuscitation
- GCS
- History
- Physical examination: assess for injuries (head, chest, abdomen, pelvis, limbs)
- Trauma X-ray series: cervical spine; chest; pelvis
- Blood profile: haematology; biochemistry; group and save or cross-match
- Catheterise for monitoring of fluid balance, if appropriate
- If indicated: CT and laparotomy.

How might you gain venous access?

- *Peripheral*: antecubital; forearm; saphenous veins
- *Peripheral venous cut-down*: great saphenous vein

- *Central*: femoral; subclavian; internal jugular veins (Seldinger technique).

Shortly after central venous line insertion, the patient becomes hypoxic, tachypnoeic and tachycardic. What might be the cause?

- Pneumothorax
- Haemothorax
- Air embolism
- Causes unrelated to central venous line insertion (fat embolus, ARDS).

If the patient arrests, what may be the cause? What would you then do?

For a tension pneumothorax, insert a large-bore cannula into the 2nd intercostal space, mid-clavicular line on the side of the suspected pneumothorax. A chest drain will then be required for definitive management.

Other reversible causes of cardiac arrest include cardiac tamponade, thromboembolism, toxins, hypoxia, hypovolaemia, hyper/hypokalaemia, and hypothermia (remember the 4Ts and 4Hs).

Acute respiratory distress syndrome (ARDS)

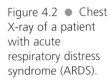 **Please refer to *Bailey and Love*, Chapter 20.**

A surgical patient develops hypoxaemia with minimal improvement on supplementary oxygen therapy. A chest X-ray shows signs of pulmonary oedema but there are no other clinical signs of heart failure.

What is the likely diagnosis?

The likely diagnosis is ARDS (non-cardiogenic pulmonary oedema) (Fig. 4.2).

Figure 4.2 ● Chest X-ray of a patient with acute respiratory distress syndrome (ARDS).

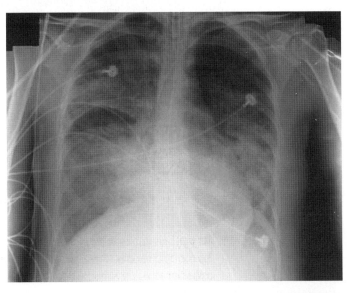

What is ARDS?

- Severe acute lung injury
- Progressive and refractory hypoxaemia
- Diffuse bilateral pulmonary infiltrates on chest X-ray
- Non-cardiac cause (normal pulmonary artery wedge pressure does not exceed 18 mmHg)
- Reduced lung compliance
- Ventilation–perfusion mismatch.

What might be causing the oedema?

Direct (pulmonary)

- Pneumonia
- Chest trauma
- Aspiration pneumonitis
- Near-drowning
- Inhalational injury.

Indirect (systemic)

- Sepsis
- Shock
- Burns
- Polytrauma
- Head injury
- Embolus (fat, air)
- Acute pancreatitis
- Cardiopulmonary bypass
- Transfusion.

How should this patient be managed?

- A – B – C – D – E
- History and physical examination
- Investigate cause
- Oxygen therapy
- Early discussion with anaesthetist and chest physiotherapist regarding ventilatory support.

What are the types of respiratory failure?

- *Type 1 respiratory failure.* Stiff lungs in ARDS causes problems with gas exchange, resulting in hypoxia. There may be compensatory hyperventilation which may lead to hypocarbia.
- *Type 2 respiratory failure.* There is a ventilatory problem, causing hypoventilation and resulting in hypercarbia as well as hypoxia. Surgical causes include head injury, stroke, respiratory depressants, trauma, epidural anaesthesia, tumour etc. Other causes include COPD and asthma.

How do you manage ARDS?

Treat the cause and support the patient:

- Intubation, high-flow fraction of inspired O_2 *(FiO$_2$)*
- Low tidal volumes, avoiding barotrauma
- 'Permissive hypercapnia' to prevent barotrauma and volutrauma
- Pressure-controlled, inverse inspiratory:expiratory ratio ventilation
- PEEP/CPAP
- Prone ventilation
- Physiotherapy
- Keep lungs dry, use inotropes to support cardiac output
- Treat sepsis
- Nutritional support
- Treat complications early
- Steroids: may prevent progression to the destructive fibrotic phase of the disease
- Consider NO, prostacyclin, surfactant (all experimental).

Fluid balance

B&L **Please refer to *Bailey and Love*, Chapter 17.**

What are the signs that a patient is dehydrated? How would you resuscitate them?

Signs are dry mucous membranes, tachycardia, reduced urine output, and drowsiness. Intravenous dextrose resuscitates and rehydrates by moving into cells.

How would you resuscitate a shocked, hypovolaemic patient?

- Colloid and blood (fluid volume is retained in the vascular compartment)
- Hartmann's solution (maintains composition of extracellular fluid when large volumes of resuscitation fluid are given).

Which fluids are good for maintenance?

- 0.9 per cent normal saline with potassium supplementation
- Hartmann's solution.

What factors determine how much fluid should be given?

- Pre-existing fluid deficit
- Maintenance fluids required
- Ongoing losses (sensible and insensible losses).

Which conditions require increased maintenance fluids?

- Pyrexia
- Ileus
- Vomiting
- High stoma output

- Fistulae
- Pancreatitis
- Polyuria (common in neurosurgical patients).

What options are there to monitor fluid balance status?
- History: patient feels thirsty
- Physical examination: assessment of mucous membranes; skin turgor; GCS; heart rate; blood pressure; jugular venous pressure (JVP); urine output (minimum 0.5 mL/kg/hour); pulse oximetry
- Blood profile: renal function; haematocrit
- Urine specific gravity
- Electrocardiogram; chest X-ray
- Central venous pressures
- Pulmonary artery flotation catheter (monitors left heart pressures and cardiac output).

What information can be gained from the pulse oximeter? Is it reliable?
Heart rate, arterial oxygen saturation and peripheral perfusion status can be determined. It is not reliable if saturation is less than 70 per cent, the patient is moving, there is venous congestion, or the patient is wearing coloured nail varnish.

Bowel obstruction

B&L   **For further reading see *Bailey and Love*, Chapter 66**
A patient presents to A&E after a laparotomy, with vomiting, absolute constipation and abdominal pain. The likely diagnosis is small bowel obstruction.

What is the most common aetiology of small bowel obstruction?
Adhesions. Other causes include hernia, strictures (e.g. Crohn's disease), tumours, gallstones.

How would you confirm the diagnosis of small bowel obstruction?
An abdominal X-ray would show central dilated loops (>3 cm diameter), valvulae conniventes.

How would you manage the patient with small bowel obstruction?
- A – B – C – D – E and fluid resuscitation
- History and physical examination
- Nil by mouth and nasogastric tube
- Catheterise
- Intravenous fluids (Hartmann's or normal saline with potassium supplementation)
- Analgesia and antiemetic.

What are common causes of large bowel obstruction, and how would you investigate it?

Tumours and strictures are the common causes.

- Abdominal X-ray and CT staging
- Contrast enema (barium/gastrograffin)
- MR staging for cancers of the rectum.

What problems can arise with patients on total parenteral nutrition?

- Line sepsis
- Pneumothorax
- Infective endocarditis
- Metabolic disturbances
- Refeeding syndrome.

Transfusion

B&L **For further reading see Bailey and Love, Chapter 2.**

Which type of packed red blood cell product can be given to a patient with blood group AB?

Any type, because group AB = universal acceptor. (Group O negative = universal donor.)

What is the volume of one unit of packed red cells? How does transfusing one unit affect the haemoglobin concentration?

Approximately 300 mL. A dose of 4 mL/kg (one pack to 70 kg adult) typically raises venous Hb concentration by about 1 g/dL.

Are there any potential problems that may arise, post-transfusion?

- Immune reactions: haemolysis
- Volume overload
- Coagulopathy: absence of clotting factors, especially V and VIII (thus supplement with fresh frozen plasma)
- Thrombocytopenia
- Hyperkalaemia (potassium leaks from packed red cells during storage)
- Hypocalcaemia (citrate is added to the packed red cell suspension to increase longevity during storage but this chelates calcium)
- Hypothermia (packed red cell blood is stored at 4°C for a shelf-life of 35 days)
- Infection with HBV, HCV, syphilis, *Yersinia*, staphylococcus.

→ Case study

You are called to see a patient being transfused who is complaining of a headache and abdominal pain, is now pyrexial and has started to drop their blood pressure. What is the diagnosis? How do you manage this patient?

The patient has suffered a haemolytic transfusion reaction. Stop the transfusion. Then:

- A – B – C – D – E and fluid resuscitation
- History and physical examination
- Blood profile: haematology (anaemia secondary to haemolysis) and biochemistry (bilirubin)
- Repeat group and save, and cross-match (Coombs' testing).

Send blood cultures in case of sepsis from contaminated blood.

Drugs

B&L   For further reading see *Bailey and Love*, Chapter 14.

What might you do to improve the circulation status of a patient in septic shock?
- Fluid resuscitation (pyrexia, with increased fluid losses though sweat)
- Inotropic agents (there is a hyperdynamic circulation with peripheral vasodilatation).

What are inotropic agents? Name a few examples.
Inotropic agents are drugs that act on alpha- and beta-adrenergic receptors causing increase in cardiac contractility and rate, and increased peripheral vascular resistance. This therefore improves cardiac output and blood pressure. Examples are dopamine, dobutamine, adrenaline and noradrenaline.

Name some sedative drugs, and how you would reverse their effects.
- Benzodiazepines (e.g. midazolam) – reverse with flumazenil
- Barbiturates (e.g. thiopentone) – no known antidote; give respiratory support
- Intravenous anaesthetic agents (e.g. propofol) – no known antidote, but short duration of action
- Inhalational anaesthetic agents (e.g. isoflurane) – reverse with pure oxygen.

Name some types of muscle relaxants.
- Depolarising agents (e.g. suxamethonium)
- Non-depolarising agents (e.g. vecuronium, atracurium – reversed by neostigmine).

Head injury

B&L   For further reading see *Bailey and Love*, Chapter 23.

A patient complains of headache and nausea, and is drowsy after a head injury. Is this significant? What would you do next?

Yes, it is significant because of possible raised intracranial pressure and the danger of reduced cerebral perfusion pressure and cerebral herniation (Monro–Kellie doctrine of fixed intracranial space) (Figs 4.3 and 4.4).

Figure 4.3 ● Normal intracranial contents are brain tissue, cerebrospinal fluid (CSF) and arterial and venous blood. During the compensation phase, CSF and venous blood volumes are reduced. When this egress of CSF and venous blood is maximal, further increases in the size of the mass lesion will cause brain herniation. (Bailey and Love, Figure 23.2, p.300.)

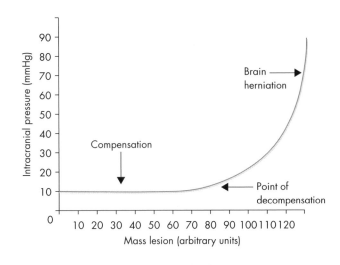

Figure 4.4 ● Brain herniation. Herniation of the cingulate gyrus under the falx cerebri is called subfalcine herniation (1). Herniation is associated with midline shift (2). Herniation of the uncus of the temporal lobe (3) is associated with compression of the ipsilateral third nerve. Central herniation (4) and tonsillar herniation (5) are associated with compression of brainstem structures. (Bailey and Love, Figure 23.3, p.300.)

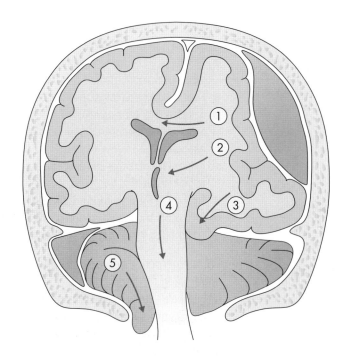

- History and physical examination
- GCS: intubate early if the clinical picture suggests deterioration to 8/15 or less
- Check for papilloedema
- Full neurological examination
- CT head scan.

What might cause raised intracranial pressure (ICP)?

- Intracranial bleeding
- Brain tumour
- Cerebral oedema
- Hydrocephalus.

Name some secondary causes of brain injury.

Primary brain injury takes place when the primary insult occurs and is considered irreversible. Secondary brain injury results from processes initiated by the primary insult that occur some time later and that may be prevented or ameliorated. Management of head injury aims to prevent secondary brain injury.

Causes of secondary brain injury include raised ICP, vasospasm, hypoxia, hypotension, hypercarbia, hyperpyrexia, hyponatraemia and other electrolyte disturbances, hyper- or hypo-glycaemia, anaemia, sepsis, raised venous pressure, and seizures.

How can a raised ICP be reduced?

- Patient positioning – nurse the patient head-up
- Avoid obstruction of venous drainage from the head (making sure cervical spine immobilisation collar is not too tight)
- Adjust $PaCO_2$ by manipulating ventilation – adjusts intracranial vessel vasoconstriction/dilatation
- Fluid balance – diuretics, mannitol etc.
- Sedation (e.g. barbiturates), with or without muscle relaxant
- Steroids (e.g. dexamethasone) – can reduce cerebral oedema around tumours
- Induced hypothermia and anticonvulsants – lower metabolic demands of brain tissue
- Tap off CSF via a ventricular catheter
- Emergency surgical evacuation of any haematoma causing mass effect – burr holes, craniotomy, decompressive craniectomy.

What emergency neurosurgical procedures may be undertaken for head injury?

- Burr hole – frontal, parietal, temporal or occipital
- Craniotomy/craniectomy
- Ventricular tap via frontal burr hole
- Elevation of compound depressed skull facture.

What are the indications for CT in head injuries?

- Falling GCS score
- Persisting neurological signs, headache, or vomiting after resuscitation
- Clinical suspicion of a fracture of the skull base: CSF rhinorrhoea/otorrhoea; Battle's sign; subconjunctival haemorrhage with no ascertainable posterior border
- Suspected penetrating head injury
- Post-traumatic seizure
- Patient has a coagulopathy (e.g. on warfarin)
- Patient is difficult to fully assess (e.g. alcohol intoxication).

What are the intracranial abnormalities that indicate urgent neurosurgical management?

- High or mixed density intracranial lesion (size and site)
- Midline shift
- Obliteration of third ventricle/basal cisterns
- Contralateral ventricular dilatation
- Intracranial air
- Subarachnoid or intraventricular haemorrhage.

Brainstem death

B&L **For further reading see *Bailey and Love*, pp.1416–1421.**

You are the specialty registrar (ST2) in General Surgery and are called at 2 am by the ST3 in ICU saying that your surgical patient is now brainstem dead. You go to ICU to review the patient.

Between the ICU ST3 and yourself, can you confirm brainstem death?

No. This can only be legally confirmed by two clinicians, one of whom is a Consultant and the other GMC registered for at least 5 years. They must also be either an intensivist, anaesthetist, neurologist or neurosurgeon.

What are the clinical criteria for brainstem death?

- Patient in an apnoeic coma (reliant entirely on mechanical ventilation due to the complete absence of spontaneous ventilation) with a GCS of 3/15
- Identification of the cause of apnoeic coma
- Exclusion of reversible causes (drugs, alcohol, hypothyroidism, uraemia, hypoglycaemia, hypothermia etc.)
- Clinical demonstration of absence of brainstem reflexes:
  - pupillary light reflex
  - corneal reflex
  - gag and cough reflex
  - vestibulo-ocular reflex (caloric testing)
  - oculo-cephalic reflexes (doll's eye manoeuvre)

- cranial motor function
- respiratory drive following a rise in $PaCO_2$ (apnoea testing).

You get a call from the organ transplantation team confirming that the patient is legally registered for organ donation. They ask you if the patient's clinical condition meets the criteria for donation. What do they mean?

■ Confirmation of brainstem death
■ No sepsis
■ No history of malignancy (except for brain tumours)
■ No history of IV drug abuse
■ HIV- and HBV-negative
■ No history of myocardial infarction (for heart donation)
■ No history of alcohol abuse (for liver donation).

Which organs may be donated?

Heart; lungs; liver; kidneys; pancreas; small bowel; bones; tendons; corneas; skin.

Patient safety and surgical skills

Who provides consent in the following clinical situations?
A 15-year-old boy requires an orchidopexy
The parent or guardian gives consent on his behalf. The procedure and its potential risks are explained to the child and the parent or guardian.

In some situations, consent for a child under 16 years of age may be obtained from the child, without their parents or legal guardian consenting on their behalf, if the child is deemed competent to understand the information and make an informed decision (termed 'Gillick competence'). However, in practice this is a situation that should be avoided if at all possible.

A 75-year-old who is unconscious and requires an emergency operation
In the case of an unconscious patient, the law recognises that it is in the patient's best interest for such an emergency treatment to go ahead. However, it is always good practice to involve the next of kin in any decision. If no next of kin is available, it is wise to obtain a colleague's agreement with the surgical procedure proposed and carefully document this in the notes.

Safe use of diathermy

What are the risks and complications of diathermy?
- Superficial burns can occur if spirit-based skin preparations are used (e.g. pooling in umbilicus).
- Diathermy burns can occur under the indifferent electrode if the plate is improperly applied.
- Arcing can occur with metal instruments and implants.
- It can interfere with pacemaker function. The two possible dangers are reprogramming of the pacemaker and myocardial burns. Avoid diathermy completely if possible, but if it is necessary use bipolar. If monopolar must be used, place the patient plate so that diathermy current flows well away from the pacemaker system and use only short bursts (<2s) at the lowest power setting possible.
- 'Channelling' effects can occur if diathermy is used on a viscus with a narrow pedicle (e.g. penis or testis).
- Sparks can ignite volatile anaesthetic gases. Use of diathermy on large bowel should therefore be avoided.

How do diathermy burns occur?
- Inadequate application of the plate electrode (see below)
- Spirit burns
- Patient touching earthed metal, such as drip stands or the metal areas of the operating table
- Faulty insulation of diathermy leads
- Inadvertent activity:
  - accidental activation of foot pedal
  - not replacing electrode in quiver after use

- accidental contact of active electrode with retractors, instruments and towel clips.
- Use of diathermy on appendages (e.g. penis, fingers and toes), so-called 'channelling effects'. Channelling effects occur because heat is produced where the current density is greatest.

Placement of the patient plate electrode

- Incorrect placement is the most common cause of accidental diathermy burns.
- It requires good contact on dry, shaved skin and kinking must be avoided.
- It is normally placed on the patient's thigh.
- The contact surface area should be at least 70 cm^2 to minimise the risk of heating.
- It should be placed away from bony prominences and scar tissue, which have poor blood supply and therefore poor heat distribution.
- It should be placed away from metallic implants (e.g. prosthetic hips).

What precautions should the surgeon take to make sure diathermy is used safely in the operating theatre?

- Wipe excess alcoholic skin preparation to dryness.
- Consider a bipolar technique.
- Avoid high-voltage modes.
- Check the patient plate electrode is used correctly (see above).
- Ensure the patient is not touching earthed metal.
- Avoid non-contact (open-circuit) activation.
- Use only enough power to achieve the desired effect.
- Check insulation (but remember that even intact insulation may fail with high voltages due to the effects of capacitance coupling).
- Do not reuse single-use electrodes.
- Place the diathermy in a safe, insulated container (quiver) when it is not being used.
- In laparoscopic surgery, keep the active electrode in full view at all times.

Laser use

What is a laser, and what are its properties?

Laser stands for light amplification by the stimulated emission of radiation. Laser light emissions are:

- collimated (a parallel output beam results in little energy loss)
- coherent (waves are all in phase, resulting in little loss of energy)
- monochromic (all of the same wave length).

The effects of a laser depend on photochemical, photomechanical and photothermal factors. Tissue penetration increases with the wavelength. Pulsing of the output can reduce thermal damage.

Figure 5.3 ● How a 'capacitance injury' may occur.

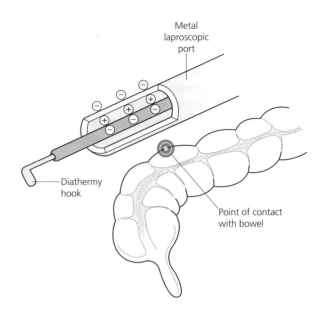

Metal laproscopic port

Diathermy hook

Point of contact with bowel

- *Theatre staff:* minimum number of individuals; avoidance of excess traffic
- *Operating personnel:* aseptic technique – hand decontamination, sterile gowns, gloves, caps, masks
- *Patient preparation:* optimise patient nutritional status; minimal pre-op hospital stay; pre-op showering; hair removal; identification of MRSA carriers; prophylactic antibiotics; mechanical bowel preparation
- *Skin preparation:* iodine or chlorhexidine; sterile wound drapes; sterile equipment
- *Surgical technique:* speed; minimise spillage; meticulous haemostasis; avoid dead space; avoid unwarranted drains; minimise foreign material; wound irrigation; choice of suture/closure material (infection rates: braided > monofilament; sutures > clips > steristrips).

What precautions would you take as a surgeon when operating on a known HIV-positive patient?

When operating on a patient whom is known, or suspected, to have an infectious condition, universal precautions should be taken in the usual manner (these are the precautions taken to protect theatre staff from infection with all cases, i.e. every patient is treated as if they are infected). Additional, special precautions should be taken.

Preoperative precautions

- Inform the anaesthetist and theatre staff.
- Use disposable instruments as far as possible.
- Put the patient **last** on the theatre list.
- Consider appropriate antibiotic prophylaxis.

Intraoperative precautions

- Use an apron, boots rather than shoes, gown, cap, mask, face visors (eye protection).
- Cover up non-intact skin surfaces.
- Consider double gloving and use of 'indicator' glove systems.
- Ensure good haemostasis throughout.
- Use diathermy rather than a scalpel.
- Ensure sharps are discarded quickly and efficiently, with no hand-to-hand passage of sharps, a 'no-touch' surgical technique when handling needles, no hand-held needles, use of blunt needles where possible, and avoiding resheathing of needles.
- Ensure theatre staff and equipment are kept to a minimum.
- Ensure spills are cleaned up meticulously.

The Pathology department should be notified in advance of infectious specimens and all infectious specimens labelled as high risk.

Postoperative precautions

- Patients are at high risk of wound infections, dehiscence and delayed healing.
- Special precautions are also used for infective cases to prevent spread of infection to other patients (e.g. MRSA, *Acinetobacter*).

How may surgical wounds be classified?

- *Clean:* an incision in which no inflammation is encountered in a surgical procedure, without a break in sterile technique, and during which the respiratory, alimentary or genitourinary tracts are not entered (e.g. thyroidectomy).
  - Infection rate is 1.5–5.1 per cent.
- *Clean–contaminated:* an incision through which the respiratory, alimentary or genitourinary tract is entered under controlled conditions but with no contamination encountered (e.g. cholecystectomy).
  - Infection rate is 7.7–10.8 per cent.
- *Contaminated:* an incision undertaken during an operation in which there is a major break in sterile technique or gross spillage from the gastrointestinal tract, or an incision in which acute, non-purulent inflammation is encountered. Open traumatic wounds that are more than 12–24 hours old also fall into this category (e.g. elective colorectal surgery).
  - Infection rate is 15.2–16.3 per cent.
- *Dirty or infected:* an incision undertaken during an operation in which the viscera are perforated or when acute inflammation with pus is encountered, and for traumatic wounds where treatment is delayed, there is faecal contamination, or devitalised tissue is present (e.g. emergency surgery for faecal peritonitis from a colonic perforation).
  - Infection rate is 28.0–40.0 per cent.

Surgical techniques

- Meticulous haemostasis at surgery, including the use of local haemostatics such as surgicel, fibrin glue and sealants.

Autologous transfusion

- Preoperative autologous blood donation
- Acute normovolaemic haemodilution
- Intraoperative and postoperative cell salvage techniques.

Day case surgery

B&L **For further reading see *Bailey and Love*, p.198.**

What are the advantages and disadvantages of day case surgery?

Advantages:

- Release of inpatient beds
- Greater efficiency of operating list scheduling
- A firm date and time for operation with reduced cancellation risk
- Reduced disruption to patients' lives
- Reduced incidence of nosocomial infections
- Cost efficacy.

Disadvantages:

- Requirement for adequate aftercare
- Experienced and trained surgical and anaesthetic staff mandatory
- Requirement for inpatient admission or readmission in cases of unexpected complications, inadequate analgesia.

What are the criteria for day case surgery?

Patient-related factors

- ASA class I or II
- Body mass index < 35
- Patient acceptability
- Psychologically suitable patient.

Surgical factors

- Operation < 1 hour duration
- An operation that is not associated with:
  - significant blood loss or fluid shifts
  - significant nausea and vomiting
  - pain that cannot be treated with simple analgesia
  - prolonged immobilisation
- An operation that has a low morbidity with a low incidence of postoperative complications.

Social factors

- Patient lives < 1 hour's drive from the unit

- Someone to drive the patient home after surgery
- A responsible adult to supervise the patient at home for the first 24/48 hours postoperatively
- Patient access to a telephone, lift (for an upper floor flat), and toilet at home.

The patient with multiple injuries: ATLS principles and practice

B&L **For further reading see *Bailey and Love*, Chapter 22.**

How would you manage a multiply injured patient who is brought to the Accident and Emergency Department following a road traffic accident?

The patient needs to be assessed according to the principles of ATLS. This involves the following:

Primary survey

- Airway with cervical spine immobilisation
- Breathing and ventilation
- Circulation with haemorrhage control
- Disability (neurological status)
- Exposure and environment.

Adjuncts to primary survey

- Monitoring tools: pulse oximetry; blood pressure; CO_2 monitor; ECG; cardiac monitor; arterial blood gases; temperature probe
- Blood tests: glucose (finger-prick test); full blood count; urea and electrolytes; amylase; clotting screen; toxicology; cross-matching; a pregnancy test for all females of child-bearing age
- Two wide-bore cannulae for intravenous fluids
- Analgesia (often neglected)
- Urinary catheter, if not contraindicated
- Nasogastric tube, if not contraindicated
- X-rays (trauma series): lateral cervical spine (including T1 vertebra), plus anteroposterior views of chest and pelvis
- Other investigations: abdominal ultrasound scan (FAST scan); diagnostic peritoneal lavage; CT scan (if patient stable).

AMPLE history

- **A**llergies
- **M**edications
- **P**ast medical and surgical history / **P**regnancy
- **L**ast meal and fluid / **L**ast tetanus
- **E**vents / **E**nvironment related to the injury.

- Perform gag reflex on each side.
- Assess the patient's voice (volume, quality) and phonation.
- Ask the patient to cough and swallow.

→ Spinal accessory (XI) nerve

- Inspect the trapezius muscle for tone and bulk. Ask the patient to shrug the shoulders and repeat against resistance.
- Inspect the sternomastoid for tone and bulk. Ask the patient to turn the head and repeat against resistance.

→ Hypoglossal (XII) nerve

- Ask the patient to protrude the tongue. Assess for symmetry, bulk, wasting or fasciculations. The tongue will deviate to the affected side.
- Assess strength on lateral deviation by asking the patient to move the tongue from side to side and then assess bulk and contraction strength.

→ Thank the patient and wash your hands

→ Summarise and offer your differential diagnosis

GCS: examination

→ Introduction and handwash

- Have the patient sitting up on the examination couch or chair.
- The GCS examination provides a reliable and objective way of recording the consciousness level of the patient. Three types of responses (eye, verbal, motor) are independently assessed.
- Ask the conscious patient whether they have any pain.

→ Inspection

General

- Look at the patient as a whole: well/unwell; pain/pain-free.
- Check the patient's prescription chart for medications (sedation and analgesia) that may alter consciousness level.

Specific

- A scoring system is used to monitor changes in the level of consciousness. The total score is the summation of the eye, verbal and motor responses.
- The range is from 3 (worst) to 15 (best).

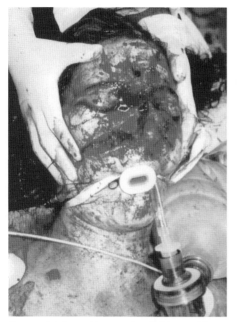

Figure 6.1.1 ● Unrestrained driver with severe craniofacial injury (courtesy of Johannesburg Hospital Trauma Unit). (Bailey and Love, Figure 22.2, p.287.)

→ Responses (GCS)

Best eye response

4 – Spontaneously
3 – To speech
2 – To pain
1 – No response

Best verbal response

5 – Orientated
4 – Confused
3 – Inappropriate responses
2 – Inappropriate sounds
1 – No response

Best motor response

6 – Obeys commands
5 – Localise to pain
4 – Withdraws from pain
3 – Flexion to pain (decorticate)
2 – Extension to pain (decerebrate)
1 – No response

→ Records

■ Pupil size: 1–8 (mm)
Pupil reaction: + = reacts; – = no reaction; c = closed eyes
■ Limb movement: normal power; mild weakness; severe weakness; spastic flexion; extension; no response.

→ Thank the patient and wash your hands

→ Summarise and offer your differential diagnosis

Peripheral nervous system: examination

→ Introduction and handwash

■ Have the patient sitting up on the examination couch or chair.
■ Expose the patient's upper and lower limbs.
■ Ask the patient whether they have any pain.
■ Remember the anatomy of the spinal cord tracts:
  • *descending pyramidal tract*: corticospinal (arm/leg weakness – upper motor neuron)
  • *descending extrapyramidal tract*: rubrospinal/vestibulospinal (ataxia)

- *spinothalamic tract*: pain and temperature sensation
- *dorsal columns*: light touch, proprioception and vibration sense
- *autonomic pathways*: bladder and sexual function.

■ Remember the spinal nerve is a mixed nerve:
- *sensory root*: specific dermatomal sensory deficit (pain, temperature, light touch, joint position sense, vibration, coordination)
- *motor root*: in lower motor neurone deficits, look for weakness, fasciculation, muscle wasting or loss of reflexes.

→ ## Inspection

General

■ Look around the bed for aids (walking, hearing).

■ Look at the patient as a whole: well/unwell; pain/pain-free.

Specific

■ Inspect the patient's muscles for wasting, hypertrophy and involuntary movements (fasciculations, choreiform movements, tremor or jerks).

■ Assess the patient's gait.

■ Perform Romberg's test.
- Ask the patient to stand with feet together, eyes open and hands by the sides. The patient should then close their eyes. Maintaining balance while standing relies on intact sensory pathways, sensorimotor integration centres and motor pathways.
- The first stage (standing with eyes open) demonstrates that at least one of the sensory pathways is intact.
- In the second stage, the visual pathway is removed by closing the eyes. If the proprioceptive pathway is intact, balance will be maintained.
- A positive Romberg test will demonstrate a sensory ataxia. This occurs with disruption in the dorsal columns of the spinal cord (tabes dorsalis – neurosyphilis), disruption of the sensory nerves (chronic inflammatory demyelinating polyradiculoneuropathy) or when there is vestibular dysfunction.

→ ## Tone

■ Ask the patient to relax and 'go floppy'.

■ Upper limb: Roll arm in clockwise and counter-clockwise directions. Perform in both limbs.

■ Lower limb: Roll leg and lift and release the patient's knee. Perform in both limbs.
- upper motor neuron lesions: 'clasp knife' spasticity and 'lead pipe' rigidity
- Parkinson's disease: 'cogwheel' rigidity.

■ Assess for clonus. Support the patient's flexed knee with one hand. Use your other hand and sharply dorsiflex the foot and sustain pressure. If positive, there will be a continued rhythmical beating of the foot.

→ Power

Table 6.1.1
Upper limb function

Movement	Root	Nerve	Muscle
Shoulder abduction	C5	Axillary	Deltoid
Elbow flexion	C5	Musculocutaneous	Biceps
Elbow flexion	C6	Radial	Brachioradialis
Elbow extension	C7	Radial	Triceps
Wrist extension	C6	Radial	Extensor carpi radialis longus
Finger extension	C7	Posterior interosseus	Extensor digitorum communis
Finger flexion	C8	Anterior interosseus	Flexor digitorum profundus (index)
Finger flexion	C8	Ulnar	Flexor digitorum profundus (ring + little)
Finger abduction	T1	Ulnar	Abductor digiti minimi
Finger abduction	T1	Median	Abductor pollicis brevis

Table 6.1.2
Cervical nerve root lesions in the upper limb

Root	C5	C6	C7	C8	T1
Sensory loss	Lateral border upper arm to elbow	Lateral forearm Thumb and index finger	Front and back of hand Middle finger	Hypothenar eminence	Axilla
Pain distribution	As above Medial scapula border	As above, especially thumb and index	As above	As above, up to elbow	Shoulder Axilla to olecranon
Motor deficit	Deltoid Supraspinatus Infraspinatus	Biceps Brachioradialis Pronators and supinators of forearm	Triceps Wrist extensors Wrist flexors Latissimus dorsi Pectoralis major	Finger flexors Finger extensors	Small muscles of hand
Reflex arc	Biceps	Supinator	Triceps	Finger	None

Table 6.1.3
Lower limb function

Movement	Root	Nerve	Muscle
Hip flexion	L2/L3	Femoral	Iliopsoas
Hip adduction	L2/L3	Obturator	Adductors
Hip extension	L4/L5	Sciatic	Gluteus maximus
Knee flexion	L5/S1	Sciatic	Hamstrings
Knee extension	L3/L4	Femoral	Quadriceps
Ankle dorsiflexion	L4/L5	Deep peroneal	Tibialis anterior
Ankle eversion	L5/S1	Superficial peroneal	Peronei
Ankle plantarflexion	S1/S2	Tibial	Gastrocnemius
Big toe extension	L5	Deep peroneal	Extensor hallucis longus

Table 6.1.4
Lumbar radiculopathy secondary to lumbar disc protrusions

	L3/L4	L4/L5	L5/S1
Disc	5%	45%	50%
Root	L4	L5	S1
Reflex	Knee	—	Ankle
Motor	Knee extension	Extensor hallucis longus Tibialis anterior	Plantar flexion
Sensory	Medial calf	Lateral calf	Lateral foot
Pain	Anterior thigh	Posterior leg	Posterior leg Ankle

- Perform isometric and isotonic testing (consult Tables 6.1.1–6.1.4).
- Assess individual muscle groups and compare each side.
- Record the MRC grading of power:
  - 5 = full power
  - 4 = against resistance
  - 3 = against gravity
  - 2 = affect of gravity removed
  - 1 = flicker of movement
  - 0 = no movement

→ Coordination

Upper limb function

- Finger–nose test: Ask the patient to hold their arm outstretched and then touch the tip of their index finger to their nose and then to your index finger. Next, move your index finger in order for the patient to touch a new target.
- Rapid alternating hand movements: Ask the patient to simulate

playing the piano. Ask the patient to place their palms upwards. The patient should then tap the upward facing palm with their palmar and then doral aspect of their fingertips from the other hand.

Lower limb function

■ Heal–shin test: Ask the patient to raise one leg at the hip and place their heel of the flexed leg on their contralateral knee and then run their heel down the anterior surface of their shin towards their ankle. Repeat the process again and in both lower limbs.

■ Heel–toe test of gait: Ask the patient to walk in a straight line in order for the heel of one foot to be in contact with toes of their other foot. Ask the patient to walk 'heel-to-toe'.

→ ## Sensation

Fine-touch function

■ Establish a baseline for fine-touch (e.g. sternal area) before examining the limbs.

■ Assess fine touch by using a small piece of cotton wool.

■ Ask the patient to close their eyes and to respond when they are touched.

■ Alter the timing of the stimulus so the patient does not anticipate the stimulus.

■ Examine the spinal segments with an anatomical system (follow the dermatomal distribution in Table 6.1.5 and Fig. 6.1.2).

■ Compare this sensation on each of the patient's limbs for symmetry. The patient should also report the quality and quantity of this sensation.

Table 6.1.5
Dermatomal distributions

Upper limb		Lower limb	
C5	Lateral arm	L1	Below inguinal ligament
C6	Thumb and index finger	L2	Middle thigh
C7	Middle finger	L3	Lower thigh
C8	Ring and small finger	L4	Medial leg and medial foot
T1	Medial arm	L5	Lateral leg and dorsal foot
		S1	Lateral foot

Pain function

■ Establish a baseline for sharpness (e.g. sternal area) before examining the limbs.

■ Assess pain by using a dedicated disposable pin.

■ Ask the patient to close their eyes and to respond when they are touched.

Figure 6.1.2 ●
Dermatomal
distribution.

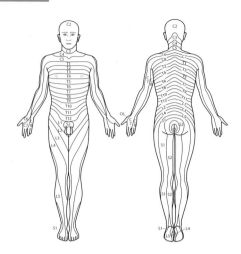

- Alter the timing of the stimulus so the patient does not anticipate the stimulus.
- Examine the spinal segments with an anatomical system (follow the dermatomal distribution in Table 6.1.5 and Fig. 6.1.2).
- Compare this sensation on each of the patient's limbs for symmetry. The patient should also report the quality and quantity of this sensation.

Temperature function

- Establish a baseline for temperature (e.g. sternal area) before examining the limbs.
- Assess temperature by using a cold and warmed tuning fork or plastic container.
- Ask the patient to close their eyes and to respond when they are touched.
- Alter the timing of the stimulus so the patient does not anticipate the stimulus.
- Examine the spinal segments with an anatomical system (follow the dermatomal distribution in Table 6.1.5 and Fig. 6.1.2).
- Compare this sensation on each of the patient's limbs for symmetry. The patient should also report the quality and quantity of this sensation.

Joint position sense (JPS) function

- Demonstrate to the patient the intended movement before examining the limbs.
- Assess JPS in the distal part of the limbs (distal interphalangeal joints of the index finger and hallux).
- Ask the patient to close their eyes and to move their distal phalanx up and down.
- Ask the patient to identify the direction of the movement.
- Compare this function on each of the patient's limbs for symmetry.

Vibration function

■ Establish a baseline for vibration (e.g. over the sternum) before examining the limbs.
■ Assess vibration by using a tuning fork (128 Hz).
■ Ask the patient to close their eyes and to respond when they are touched.
■ Alter the timing of the stimulus so the patient does not anticipate the stimulus.
■ In the upper limbs, use the interphalangeal joint of the forefinger, wrist, elbow or shoulder. In the lower limbs, use the big toes, ankle (medial malleolus), tibial tuberosity or iliac crest.
■ Compare this sensation on each of the patient's limbs for symmetry.

Two-point discrimination function

■ Assess discrimination by using an opened paperclip.
■ Ask the patient to close their eyes and to respond when they are touched.
■ Alter the timing of the stimulus so the patient does not anticipate the stimulus.
■ Apply the opened paperclip to the digits and ask whether one or two stimuli are felt.

→ ## Reflexes

■ Perform deep tendon and superficial reflexes. If the reflex is absent, you may be able to enhance the reflex with reinforcement.
■ Ensure the patient is in a position of comfort with the limbs relaxed.
■ Tap the tendon of the muscle with a tendon hammer and observe for muscle contraction.
■ Record the grading:
  • 4+ = hyperactive with clonus
  • 3+ = hyperactive
  • 2+ = normal
  • 1+ = hypoactive
  • 0 = no reflex

Specific reflexes

■ Tendon reflex: see Table 6.1.6.

Table 6.1.6
Tendon reflexes

Upper limb	Lower limb
Biceps (C5, musculocutaneous nerve)	Patellar (L3–L4, femoral nerve)
Brachioradialis (C6, radial nerve)	Achilles (S1–S2, tibial nerve)
Triceps (C7, radial nerve)	

- Finger jerks (C8)
- Hoffmann reflex: Hold the patient's middle finger (distal interphalangeal joint) and briskly flick the patient's finger tip down and examine the patient's thumb for movement
- Pectoral reflex
- Deltoid reflex
- Plantar response: Apply a blunt implement to the lateral border of the patient's sole. A normal reflex is plantar flexion of the hallux with flexion and adduction of the other toes
- Abdominal response
- Cremasteric reflex.

→ Thank the patient and wash your hands

→ Summarise and offer your differential diagnosis

Median nerve: examination

→ Introduction and handwash

- Have the patient in a comfortable position on the examination couch or chair.
- Obtain adequate exposure.
- Ask the patient whether they have any pain.

→ Look

General
- Look around the bed for aids (wrist splints).
- Look at the patient as a whole: well/unwell; pain/pain-free.
- Look for signs of endocrine causes (acromegaly, myxoedema), connective tissue disease (rheumatoid arthritis), fluid retention (congestive cardiac failure, pregnancy) and trauma.

Specific
- Inspect the following structures:
  - skin: carpal tunnel decompression scars; pulp atrophy; cigarette burns
  - muscle: wasting of thenar eminence; flexors in the forearm; the short flexors; abductor and opponens of the thumb; the lumbricals to the index and middle finger
  - bone: Simian thumb.

→ Feel

- Ask the patient whether they are in pain before you begin.
- Palpate for pain in the hand.

- Palpate the median nerve at the wrist (superficial site).
- Test sensation over the tip of the patient's index finger.
- Test sensation over the thenar eminence.

→ **Move**

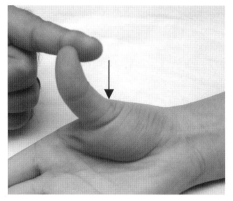

Figure 6.1.3 ● Testing the power of the abductor pollicis brevis supplied by the median nerve. (Bailey and Love, Figure 31.17, p.439.)

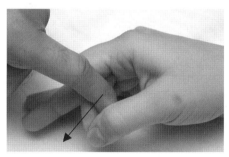

Figure 6.1.4 ● Test for the flexor pollicis longus supplied by the anterior interosseus nerve. (Bailey and Love, Figure 31.14, p.439.)

- Test the LOAF muscles (**l**ateral two lumbricals, **o**pponens pollicis, **a**bductor pollicis brevis, **f**lexor pollicis brevis).
- Abductor pollicis brevis: Ask the patient to place their hand on the examination couch, palm facing up and to point their thumb to the ceiling. Ask the patient to resist you pushing the thumb down (Fig. 6.1.3). Feel simultaneously for muscle contraction in the thenar eminence.
- Opposition (thumb to each finger).
- 'OK' sign test (tests flexor pollicis longus (FPL) thumb, flexor digitorum profundus (FDP) index finger; anterior interosseous branch of median nerve) (Fig. 6.1.4). Try to break the circle between their thumb and index finger.
- FPL: Hold the base of the thumb and ask the patient to bend the tip of their thumb.
- FDP: Fix the proximal interphalangeal joint (PIPJ) and isolate the distal interphalangeal joint (DIPJ). Then ask the patient to bend the tip of their finger (Fig. 6.1.5a).
- Flexor digitorum superficialis: Hold the other fingers down in extension to eliminate the FDP and then ask the patient to flex their finger (Fig. 6.1.5b).

(a) 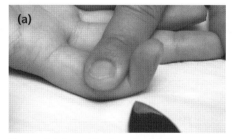   **(b)**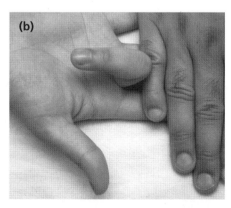

Figure 6.1.5 ● Testing the (a) flexor digitorum profundus, and (b) flexor digitorum superficialis. (Bailey and Love, Figures 31.13a and 31.13b, p.438.)

- Ask the patient to make a fist (look for the 'Benediction sign') and inspect the volar forearm for contraction of palmaris longus and flexor carpi radialis. (Make a tight fist and flex at wrist to contract forearm muscles.)
- Ask the patient to flex their wrist and look for ulnar deviation/adduction (unopposed action of flexor carpi ulnaris due to weak forearm flexors).
- Assess pronator teres: Extend the patient's elbow and pronate against resistance. You may also assess this by shaking the patient's hand and asking them to push against you.

→ Special tests

- Functional assessment:
  - power grip
  - pincer grip (pick up a coin or key)
  - button and unbutton shirt
  - hold a pen and write.
- Tinel's sign: Percuss over the median nerve from the top of the forearm down to the centre of the palm and ask the patient if they feel paraesthesia over the median nerve distribution.
- Phalen's test: Hold the patient's wrists in maximum flexion for >60 seconds and ask the patient if they feel paraesthesia over the median nerve distribution.

→ Complete the median nerve examination

- Perform a full neurological assessment of the upper and lower limbs.
- Perform a full vascular examination of the upper and lower limbs.
- Examine the joint above (shoulder and cervical spine).
- Assess the impact of the joint condition on the patient's life.
- Request nerve conduction studies.
- Consider imaging of the cervical spine (radiographs, MRI scan).
- Assess the patient's fitness for surgery.

→ Thank the patient and wash your hands

→ Summarise and offer your differential diagnosis

Radial nerve: examination

→ Introduction and handwash

- Have the patient in a comfortable position on the examination couch or chair.
- Obtain adequate exposure.
- Ask the patient whether they have any pain.

→ Look

General

■ Look around the bed for aids (wrist splints).

■ Look at the patient as a whole: well/unwell; pain/pain-free.

Specific

■ Inspect the following structures:
  • skin: scars, pulp atrophy, cigarette burns
  • muscle: wasting of posterior forearm muscles (extensors)
  • bone: wrist drop and fractures of the humeral shaft.

■ Ask the patient to place their hands behind their head and check the elbows for scars (head radius fracture) and wasting of triceps muscles.

■ Ask the patient to lift their hand off the examination couch and inspect for a wrist drop.

→ Feel

■ Ask the patient whether they are in pain before you begin.

■ Palpate for pain in the hand.

■ Test sensation over the anatomical snuffbox.

■ Test sensation over the first dorsal web space.

■ Test sensation over the back of the forearm.

→ Move

■ Test extension of the triceps muscle (high lesions).

■ Test brachioradialis: Flex the elbow in mid-prone position against resistance.

■ Test supinator: Extend the elbow and supinate against resistance. Test this by holding their hand with your opposite hand; i.e. grip their right hand with your left hand and grip their left hand with your right hand. Ask them to push against you.

■ Ask them to cock their wrist back against resistance (wrist extension).

■ Test finger extension: Ask the patient to keep their fingers straight and stop you bending their fingers.

■ Extensor pollicis longus: Perform the retropulsion test. Ask the patient to put their hand on the examination couch, palm down, and lift their thumb into the air against resistance.

→ Special tests

■ Functional assessment:
  • power grip
  • pincer grip (pick up a coin or key)
  • button and unbutton shirt
  • hold a pen and write.

→ Complete the radial nerve examination

- Perform a full neurological assessment of the upper and lower limbs.
- Perform a full vascular examination of the upper and lower limbs.
- Examine the joint above (shoulder and cervical spine).
- Assess the impact of the joint condition on the patient's life.
- Request nerve conduction studies. Consider a radiograph of the humerus and radiograph and/or MRI scan of the cervical spine.
- Assess the patient's fitness for surgery.

→ Thank the patient and wash your hands

→ Summarise and offer your differential diagnosis

Ulnar nerve: examination

→ Introduction and handwash

- Have the patient in a comfortable position on the examination couch or chair.
- Obtain adequate exposure.
- Ask the patient whether they have any pain.

→ Look

General
- Look around the bed for aids (wrist splints).
- Look at the patient as a whole: well/unwell; pain/pain-free.

Specific
- Inspect the following dorsum surface structures:
  - skin: pulp atrophy; scars; cigarette burns; brittle nails
  - muscle: wasting 1st dorsal web space; interosseous (Fig. 6.1.6); dorsal guttering
  - bone: 'claw hand'
- Inspect the following palmar surface structures:
  - skin: as above
  - muscle: wasting hypothenar eminence (Fig. 6.1.6); wasting medial forearm muscles
  - bone: ask the patient to lay their hand flat down on the table to assess any fixed flexion deformity ('table-top test')
- Inspect the upper limbs: Ask the patient to place their hands behind their head. Check the elbows for scars around the medial epicondyle/forearm/wrist and check elbow for cubitus valgus (tardy ulnar syndrome).

→ Feel

- Palpate along the ulnar nerve behind the patient's medial epicondyle and over the wrist joint.

- Test sensation over the tip of the little and ring fingers (volar surface).
- Turn hands over and test the dorsal cutaneous branch of ulnar nerve (given off proximal to the wrist).

→ ## Move

- First dorsal interosseous: resisted abduction of index finger and palpate the 1st dorsal web space.
- Abductor digiti minimi: Repeat the same with the little finger.
- Finger adductors (palmar interossei): Hold a piece of paper in between the patient's fingers and ask them to try to stop you from pulling the paper away.

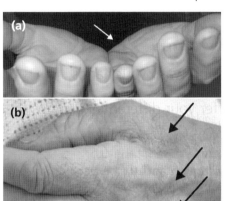

- Finger abductors (dorsal interossei): Ask the patient to spread fingers apart and stop you from pushing them together. Ask the patient to put their hands together palms up and little fingers touching, and then push the little fingers together.
- Ulnar ½ FDP: Ask the patient to bend the tip of their little finger at the DIPJ.
- Flexor carpi ulnaris (FCU) and ulnar ½ FDP: Ask the patient to make a fist (grip hard with wrist flexion). Examine for muscle contraction.
- FCU (wrist flexion and ulnar deviation at the wrist): Ask the patient to flex and adduct their wrist. Note when FCU is paralysed: flexion at the wrist joint will result in abduction.

Figure 6.1.6 ● Clinical signs of ulnar neuropathy. (a) Hypothenar eminence wasting. (b) Interosseous muscle wasting. (Bailey and Love, Figures 34.41a and 34.41b, p.502.)

→ ## Special tests

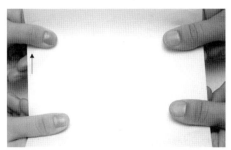

Figure 6.1.7 ● Froment's sign. The arrow illustrates the flexed posture of the thumb interphalangeal joint, indicating weakness of the adductor pollicis muscle innervated by the ulnar nerve. (Bailey and Love, Figure 31.16, p.439.)

- Functional assessment:
  - power grip
  - pincer grip (pick up a coin or key)
  - button and unbutton shirt
  - hold a pen and write
- Froment's sign (Fig. 6.1.7): Ask the patient to grasp a piece of paper between their thumb and index finger (using both hands). Try to pull paper away. Note if there is flexing of the terminal phalanx as you pull away. This test assesses adductor pollicis; in ulnar nerve palsy, the FPL flexes the IPJ to compensate.

■ Peripheral stigmata of gastrointestinal disease, such as koilonychia, angular cheilitis and glossitis (Plummer–Vinson syndrome), or features of the CREST syndrome

■ Neck examination, noting the presence of any neck lumps (e.g. pharyngeal pouch) and checking for cervical lymphadenopathy and supraclavicular lymphadenopathy – Virchow's node (Troisier's sign)

■ Abdominal examination, checking for masses, ascites, hepato-splenomegaly

■ Neurological examination (a variety of neurological abnormalities will be associated with dysphagia of neuromuscular origin)

■ Full ear, nose and throat (ENT) examination including fibreoptic laryngoscopy.

→ Investigations

Blood tests

■ *Haematology* – full blood count + iron studies + erythrocyte sedimentation rate (ESR):
  • anaemia (malignancy, Plummer–Vinson)
  • serum iron + total binding capacity + ferritin (Plummer--Vinson, GI bleed)
  • ESR (malignancy, scleroderma)

■ *Biochemistry*:
  • urea and electrolytes (dehydration)
  • liver function tests (liver metastases)

■ *Immunology*:
  • autoantibody screen (scleroderma).

Radiology

■ *Chest X-ray* (antero-posterior and lateral):
  • thyroid goitre extension; left atrial enlargement; tumours; foreign body; aspiration; achalasia (air-fluid level behind heart); thoracic aortic aneurysm

■ *Barium swallow* (in the absence of absolute dysphagia otherwise there is a risk of aspiration)
  • motility disorder (e.g. achalasia); pharyngeal pouch (oesophago-gastro-duodenoscopy (OGD) risks perforation); benign/malignant stricture; external compression; reflux

■ *CT of thorax*: staging of tumour.

OGD +/− biopsy and *H. pylori* status

■ *Diagnostic*: malignant stricture (tumour); benign peptic stricture; oesophagitis (inflammatory/infective); achalasia; foreign body

■ *Therapeutic*: balloon dilatation

■ *Surveillance*: Barrett's oesophagus (pre-malignant).

Specific investigations

- Oesophageal endoluminal ultrasound (staging of oesophageal carcinoma)
- Bronchoscopy/mediastinoscopy (assessment of invasion of oesophageal carcinoma)
- Liver ultrasound (staging of carcinoma)
- Laparoscopy (staging of carcinoma)
- Oesophageal manometry (oesophageal spasm)
- 24-hour oesophageal pH monitoring (oesophageal reflux).

Lump in the neck: history taking

You are a junior doctor on Mr Jones' ENT team. Mr Jones has asked you to clerk a new patient in the outpatient clinic. The GP referral letter is attached. After you have taken the history you will be asked to present it to one of the examiners as though he or she were the Consultant.

Drs S Green and H Brown
1 Grange Road
London

The Consultant ENT Surgeon
St Peter's Hospital
Edinburgh

Dear —

Re: George Latimer, 16 Kings Road, London

I would be grateful if you could see this 70-year-old man who came to us with a lump in the neck.

Yours sincerely

Dr H.Brown

Take a standard focused surgical history (presenting complaint, history presenting complaint, past medical history, drug history and allergies, social history, family history, systemic enquiry), but in particular enquire about the following:

- Age
- Site of lump
- Single or multiple
- Onset, duration and developmental time course – congenital versus acquired
- Presence or absence of pain

- Associated symptoms – dysphagia; dysphonia; odynophagia; referred otalgia; globus sensation; cough; haemoptysis; weight loss; symptoms of thyroid dysfunction; sore throat; intraoral diseases such as tooth decay
- Personal habits/risk factors – smoking, alcohol, betel nuts etc.
- Previous radiation or surgery
- Systemic symptoms – fever; night sweats; pruritus; anorexia; malaise
- Family history and TB contacts
- Foreign travel and risk factors for HIV infection.

Lump in the neck: examination

The same approach can be used for any skin lesion in the head and neck region.

→ Introduction

- Introduce yourself to the patient.
- Obtain consent.
- Obtain adequate exposure.
- Check whether the patient has any pain.
- Wash hands.

→ Inspection

After determining the number of lumps, apply the rule of Ss: site; size; shape; surface/smoothness; skin overlying; surroundings; special characteristics.

Site (anatomical triangle neck or level in the neck)
The borders of the anterior triangle are the anterior border of the sternocleidomastoid muscle, the ramus of the mandible and the midline. The borders of the posterior triangle are the posterior border of sternocleidomastoid, the middle one-third of the clavicle and the anterior border of the trapezius muscle.

An alternative approach is to state which level of the neck the lump is situated in, according to the Memorial Sloan–Kettering Classification (Fig. 6.2.1):

- Level 1 = submental (Ia) and submandibular (Ib) areas
- Level 2 = upper third sternocleidomastoid
- Level 3 = middle third sternocleidomastoid
- Level 4 = lower third sternocleidomastoid
- Level 5 = posterior triangle
- Level 6 = pretracheal and prelaryngeal areas.

Size
A × B centimetres.

Figure 6.2.1 ●
Oncological levels in
the neck

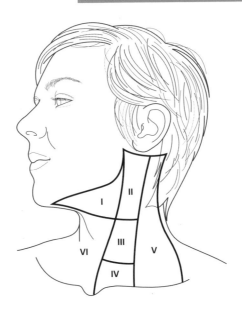

Shape
Hemispherical, lobulated.

Surface and smoothness
Identify overlying punctum and assess for a smooth/bosselated surface.

Skin overlying the lump
- Skin changes
- Skin colour
- Scars (taking care not to miss any faint tracheostomy or thyroidectomy scars)
- Evidence of previous radiotherapy.

Surroundings
Other lumps or satellite nodules?

Special characteristics
Moves with swallowing; protrusion of tongue; pulsatility.

→ Palpation

- Tenderness (before touching the lump, check with the patient whether it is tender)
- Temperature (using the back of the hand, which is more sensitive)
- Consistency: soft; firm; hard; bony hard
- Edge: diffuse versus defined
- Fluctuance: in two planes at right-angles to each other (Paget's sign).

Relationships

Try to ascertain which layer the lump is in.

- To determine its relationship to the skin, assess whether you can pinch the skin overlying the lump, or whether you can move the skin over it. If either of these is the case, the lump lies deep of the skin. Alternatively, if the lump moves with the skin, it lies within the skin.
- For skin lesions, assess whether it is flush with the skin, or raised.
- To determine the relationship of the lump to underlying muscles (e.g. sternocleidomastoid), ask the patient to tense/contract the muscle.
  - Test for mobility/fixity of the lump at rest in two orthogonal planes.
  - Then ask the patient to contract the underlying muscle.
  - Assess whether the lump is more or less prominent.
  - Assess whether the lump is more or less mobile with the muscle contracted (in two planes).

Regional lymph nodes

Never forget to assess the regional lymph node status.

Extra tests (if indicated)

Pulsatility; compressibility; thrill; transillumination; expansility; cough impulse; reducibility.

Normal structures

Palpate the normal structures of the neck – the hyoid bone, thyroid prominence of laryngeal cartilage, laryngeal cartilage, cricoid cartilage and trachea. Gently displace the larynx from side to side and feel for the normal laryngeal crepitus as the laryngeal cartilaginous framework is moved over the prevertebral muscle and fascia (this is lost in postcricoid tumours and in retropharyngeal abscesses – Trotter's sign).

→ ## Key insider's tip

As a general rule:

- If the lump retains mobility and is more prominent when underlying muscle is contracted = *lump is superficial to muscle.*
- If the lump is more prominent but less mobile when underlying muscle is contracted = *lump is attached to fascia or superficial surface of muscle.*
- If the lump is less mobile and less prominent when underlying muscle is contracted = *lump is within muscle.*
- If the lump is less mobile and less prominent when underlying muscle is contracted = *lump is deep to muscle.*

The one **exception** to this general rule occurs when there is a defect in the muscle. In such cases, although the lump arises in (or deep) to the muscle, it appears more prominent when the muscle is contracted (e.g. ruptured muscle fibres as in a torn long head of biceps, incisional hernias, divarication of the rectus sheath).

→ ## Percussion

Percussion may be useful in defining whether a goitre has retrosternal extension.

→ ## Auscultation

Listen for bruits (e.g. Graves' goitre, carotid artery aneurysm, chemodectoma).

→ ## Cervical lymphadenopathy

If the case is cervical lymphadenopathy, do not forget to check the drainage sites (Fig. 6.2.2). This will necessitate a complete ENT examination including examination of the postnasal space, oral cavity, oropharynx and fibreoptic laryngoscopy. In addition, offer to check other sites for lymphadenopathy (axilla, epitrochlear and inguinal regions, spleen, liver etc.), which may become involved, for instance in lymphoma and infections such as EBV.

→ ## Thank the patient and wash your hands

→ ## Summarise and offer your differential diagnosis

Figure 6.2.2 ●
Lymphatic drainage
and distribution.

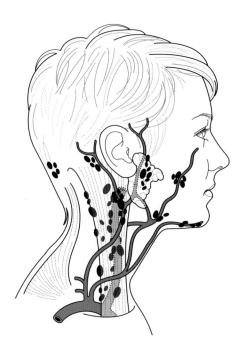

Neck swellings: differential diagnosis

See Table 6.2.1.

Table 6.2.1
Differential diagnosis of neck swellings

Midline neck swelling	Lateral neck swelling
Sebaceous cyst	Sebaceous cyst
Lipoma	Lipoma
Thyroglossal duct cyst	Cervical lymph node
Solitary nodule of thyroid isthmus	Thyroid gland enlargement
Pyramidal thyroid lobe	Branchial cyst
Dermoid cyst	Carotid body tumour
Subhyoid bursae	Pharyngeal pouch
Plunging ranula	Cystic hygroma
Pretracheal, prelaryngeal (level VI) lymph node	
Chondroma of the thyroid cartilage or larynx	

→ ## Multiple lumps

- Lymph nodes (invariably)
- Cold abscess (TB, actinomycosis).

→ ## Single lumps

Superficial

- Sebaceous cyst
- Lipoma
- Dermoid cyst
- Abscess.

Deep
See Table 6.2.2.

Table 6.2.2
Deep single lumps in the neck region

	Anterior triangle	Posterior triangle
Does not move with swallowing	Submandibular swelling Parotid swelling Branchial cyst Carotid body tumour Carotid artery aneurysm Sternomastoid 'tumour' Lymph node/cold abscess Laryngocele Chondroma	Cystic hygroma (lymphangioma) Pharyngeal pouch Cervical rib Subclavian artery aneurysm Tumour of clavicle Lymph node/cold abscess
Moves with swallowing	Thyroglossal duct cyst Thyroid gland Thyroid isthmus lymph node	

→ **The triple assessment**

If you are asked how you would manage any neck lump, the answer is always triple assessment, namely:

- **History and clinical examination**
- **Imaging:**
  - ultrasound scan
  - CT scan
  - MRI scan
  - radionucleotide scan
- **Fine-needle aspiration cytology/biopsy**.

Thyroid status: history taking

→ Local pressure symptoms

- Neck lumps: duration; change in size with time etc.
- Pain
- Dysphagia
- Stridor/dyspnoea
- Hoarseness
- Cosmesis.

→ Questions about thyroid status

- Are you taking any medications?
- Have you had any thyroid operations, or radioiodine treatments?
- Are you affected by temperature? Do you prefer hot or cold?
- Have you lost or gained weight?
- Do you have constipation or diarrhoea?
- How is your appetite?
- Do you get palpitations?
- Have your periods changed?
- Have you noticed any change in your appearance/face?
- Have you become more anxious?
- Has your skin/hair changed?
- Do you have any problems with your eyes (protruding, difficulty closing eyelids, pain secondary to exposure keratitis, double vision)?

Thyroid status: examination

→ Introduction

- Introduce yourself to the patient.
- Obtain consent.
- Obtain adequate exposure.

- Check whether the patient has any pain.
- Wash hands.

→ ## Inspection

- Perform a *general survey*. Observe the patient's demeanour: are they anxious and fidgety, suggesting thyrotoxicosis, or are they slow and lethargic, suggesting hypothyroidism? Is the patient thin or fat?

→ ## Palpation

Hands

- Fine tremor (place a piece of paper on the patient's outstretched arms, palms facing down and the fingers extended and separated)
- Thyroid acropachy (a form of nail clubbing)
- Onycholysis (separation of the nail from the nail bed)
- Palmar erythema
- Warm, moist, sweaty palms
- Pulse (tachycardia, atrial fibrillation)
- Vitiligo.

Eyes

- Is there lid retraction (upper lid higher than normal, lower lid in correct position)?
- Lid lag: Gently restrain the patient's head to prevent movement and ask the patient to follow your finger with their eyes as you lower it slowly from above. Do not do this in a rapid fashion. Lid lag occurs when the upper lid does not keep pace with the eyeball and occurs because of spasm of the smooth muscle in the upper eyelid secondary to increased sympathetic tone in thyrotoxicosis.
- Proptosis/exophthalmos: Look from in front, the side and from above; the sclera is visible below or all around the iris (Fig. 6.2.3).
- Is there chemosis?
- Look for ophthalmoplegia (eye movements).
- Look for optic nerve involvement (visual acuity).

Mouth

- Check for a for a lingual thyroid.

Neck

- Examine the thyroid gland itself.

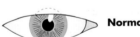
Normal

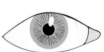
Mild exophthalmos
Sclera visible below the inferior limbus

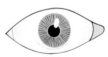
Severe exophthalmos
Sclera visible all round the iris

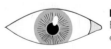
Lid retraction
Elevation of the upper eyelid

Figure 6.2.3 ● Exophthalmos versus lid retraction.

Legs

■ Check reflexes and look for evidence of pretibial myxoedema.
■ Ask the patient to stand up with their arms across their chest. Look for proximal myopathy which can occur in hypothyroidism or hyperthyroidism.

→ Assessment of thyroid status

See Table 6.2.3.

Table 6.2.3
Assessment of thyroid status

	Hyperthyroid	Hypothyroid
General	Restlessness, anxiety, weight loss, intolerance to heat	Dull, mental lethargy, intolerance to cold, brittle hair
Hands	Nails (acropachy, onycholysis), palms (sweaty, warm, palmar erythema), fine tremor, pulse (tachycardic, atrial fibrillation)	Palms (dry, rough, inelastic, cold, pale), pulse (bradycardic), carpal tunnel (positive Tinel's sign)
Eyes	Lid lag, lid retraction, exophthalmos/proptosis, ophthalmoplegia, chemosis	Periorbital puffiness, loss of outer one-third of eyebrows
Neck	Goitre, scars	Goitre, scars
Reflexes	Brisk	Delayed ankle jerks
Legs and skin	Pretibial myxoedema, vitiligo	

→ Thank the patient and wash your hands

→ Summarise and offer your differential diagnosis

Thyroid: examination

→ Introduction

■ Introduce yourself to the patient.
■ Obtain consent.
■ Obtain adequate exposure:
 • Position the chair well away from the wall so that you can get easily behind the patient to examine their neck.
 • Ask the patient to undo top buttons to expose the upper chest so that you do not miss a midline sternotomy scar (from retrosternal goitre surgery) or distended/engorged veins on the chest wall (superior vena cava obstruction).
■ Check whether the patient has any pain.
■ Wash hands.

→ Inspection

General

- Look at the patient as a whole for thyroid status: scars; tremor; myxoedema; wasting; periorbital puffiness; eye signs; swellings; asymmetry.
- Ask for a glass of water if there is not one visible.
- Assess hoarseness of the voice by asking the patient to count from 1 to 10.
- Ask them to take a deep breath in and listen for stridor.

Neck

Inspect the neck from the front, sides and back.

- Are there any obvious neck swellings or visible scars? Comment if the lump is in the anterior or posterior triangle.
- Ask the patient to open the mouth and stick out the tongue. If the swelling is a thyroglossal duct cyst, the upward tug when the patient protrudes their tongue is unmistakable. Note that the mouth must be open at the commencement of the test when the swelling is grasped. You may check for a lingual thyroid simultaneously at the base of the tongue while the patient's mouth is open.
- Ask the patient to take a sip of water, hold it in their mouth and swallow when you instruct them to, with their chin slightly elevated. Does the lump move with swallowing? If it does, it implies the swelling is thyroid-related.

→ Palpation

Explain to the patient what you are about to do and then move behind them. Ask again if it is tender.

- Palpate from behind, but look at the patient's face when you start to press on the thyroid for signs of discomfort.
- Slightly flex the patient's head. Put one hand flat on one lobe and push it towards the midline. This will make the other side more prominent. Check for tenderness and temperature.
- Ask the patient to swallow again. This time ask yourself whether you can get below the thyroid gland when the patient swallows. If you can, it excludes retrosternal extension.
- Note:
  - size of goitre
  - consistency (soft, firm, hard; uniform or varied)
  - single, diffuse or multiple swellings
  - surface smooth or nodular (any prominent nodules?)
- Also check mobility and relation to surroundings (skin, trachea, muscle and carotid artery) for fixity, displacement and infiltration:
  - Gently pinch the skin over the thyroid to check for fixity.

- Check for fixation to the trachea (in two planes) and for tracheal displacement/deviation.
- Check the relationship of the gland to the sternocleidomastoid muscle (ask the patient to look to one side and then gently push their chin down on the volar aspect of your wrist).
  - Assess the carotid artery pulsations (Berry's sign).
- Examine regional lymph nodes: submental, submandibular, deep cervical chain including the jugulodigastric group, supraclavicular, superficial cervical chain, pre- and post-auricular, occipital, pre-tracheal and pre-laryngeal groups.

→ Percussion

Percuss from the sternum upwards to check for retrosternal extension.

→ Auscultation

Auscultate for a thyroid bruit, while the patient holds his or her breath.

→ Further considerations

- Assess the patient's thyroid status and ask him/her some questions.
- Offer to check the patient's vocal cords by flexible laryngoscopy.
- Offer to perform Pemberton's test/sign. Ask the patient to elevate their arms above their head for one minute and look for congestion, cyanosis, stridor, and distended neck veins, as a sign of a large retrosternal goitre.

→ Thank the patient and wash your hands

→ Summarise and offer your differential diagnosis

Thyroid goitre: differential diagnosis

→ Simple goitres

- Physiological: pregnancy; pubertal; lactation; menstruation
- Pathological: iodine deficiency; goitrogens
- Multinodular.

→ Inflammatory

- Thyroiditis (Hashimoto's, de Quervain's, Riedel's).

→ Neoplastic

- Papillary
- Follicular/Hurthle
- Anaplastic

- Medullary
- Lymphoma.

→ Toxic

- Graves' goitre
- Solitary toxic adenoma/nodule
- Multinodular goitre (Plummer's disease).

→ Rare

- TB
- Sarcoid
- Amyloid
- HIV
- Lithium
- Amiodarone
- Syphilis.

→ The solitary thyroid nodule

The differential diagnosis includes the following:
- Simple thyroid cyst
- Adenoma/simple hyperplastic nodule
- Prominent nodule in a multinodular goitre
- Enlarged lobe (e.g. Hashimoto's thyroiditis)
- Haemorrhage into a cyst/nodule
- Carcinoma (primary or rarely secondary).

Parotid: examination

Bear in mind that you may be asked to examine the neck, and to pass this station you would be expected to spot a lump in the tail of the parotid gland.

→ Introduction

- Introduce yourself to the patient.
- Get consent.
- Obtain adequate exposure.
- Check whether the patient has any pain.
- Wash hands.

→ Inspection

- Inspect both sides.
- Look carefully for scars. The Blair incision is most often used, so demonstrate to the examiners you are looking carefully in front of the tragus, in the preauricular skin crease, and around the earlobe. If necessary, carefully lift up the earlobe.

→ Palpation

■ Check whether it is tender before proceeding.
■ Define the characteristics of the lump, as you would for any other lump.
■ Ask the patient to tense the underlying masseter muscle by getting them to clench their jaw; test for fixity.
■ Check the regional lymph node status. If you suspect the lump is a preauricular lymph node, examine the face and scalp carefully for a primary site of infection or neoplasia.

The oral cavity/oropharynx

■ Check the parotid duct (Stensen's duct) which lies opposite the upper second molar teeth (for pus, calculi etc.). Try to express pus out the parotid duct by gently massaging the gland and looking inside the oral cavity at the duct orifice.
■ Check the oropharynx for evidence of medialisation of the tonsils from a deep parotid lobe tumour, or a tumour sited in the parapharyngeal space.
■ Offer to bimanually palpate the parotid gland (feeling the duct and the gland). However, its clinical value is limited compared with examination of the submandibular gland because the parotid lies behind the anterior edge of the masseter muscle and the vertical ramus of the mandible.

Integrity of the facial (VII) nerve

Ask the patient to 'raise their eyebrows', 'shut their eyes tight', 'blow out their cheeks', 'whistle', 'show you their teeth', 'grimace'; and check taste sensation with respect to the anterior two-thirds of the tongue.

→ Further considerations

■ Check the contralateral side.
■ Test sensation around the angle of the mandible and the earlobe if the patient has had a parotidectomy (great auricular nerve injury).
■ Offer a full ENT examination.

→ Differential diagnosis

Bear in mind that not every lump in the parotid region is a parotid gland swelling. When trying to formulate a differential diagnosis, try to think what structures are in the immediate vicinity of the swelling:
■ Skin (sebaceous cyst, fungating squamous cell carcinoma)
■ Subcutaneous tissue (lipoma, dermoid cyst)
■ Muscle (masseter muscle hypertrophy)
■ Facial nerve (neuroma)
■ Lymphatics (preauricular lymph node)
■ Bone (winging of mandible, prominent transverse process atlas/axis)

■ Salivary tissue (tumours within the parotid gland itself, which may be benign or malignant).

In summary, for a lesion in the parotid region, do not forget to:
■ Check the regional lymph node status.
■ Check the integrity of the facial nerve.
■ Look in the mouth.

→ Thank the patient and wash your hands

→ Summarise and offer your differential diagnosis

Submandibular swelling: examination

→ Introduction
■ Introduce yourself to the patient.
■ Obtain consent.
■ Obtain adequate exposure.
■ Check whether the patient has any pain.
■ Wash hands.

→ Inspection
Inspect both sides carefully for scars and evidence of marginal mandibular nerve weakness.

→ Palpation
■ Check whether it is tender before proceeding.
■ Define the characteristics of the lump, as you would for any other lump.
■ To determine the relationship of the swelling to the mylohyoid muscle, ask the patient to tense the floor of the mouth (by asking the patient to push their tongue against the roof of the mouth). To determine the relationship to the sternocleidomastoid muscle, ask the patient to contract this muscle.

Inside the mouth
■ Check the submandibular (Wharton's) duct orifice under the tongue (for pus, calculi etc.)
■ Look for evidence of dental infection, or a primary carcinoma in the mouth (submental and submandibular lymph nodes drain the oral cavity).

Bimanual palpation of the submandibular gland
■ Before proceeding, ask for gloves. Generally, submandibular glands are ballottable whereas submandibular lymph nodes are not.

■ Try to express pus out of the submandibular duct by gently massaging the gland and looking inside the oral cavity at the duct orifice.

Tongue
Test tongue sensation (lingual nerve) and mobility (hypoglossal nerve) for malignant infiltration of nerves.

Regional lymph nodes
Check regional lymph node status.

→ Further considerations

■ Check the contralateral side and the parotid glands.
■ Offer a full ENT examination.

→ Thank the patient and wash your hands

→ Summarise and offer your differential diagnosis

Trunk and thorax

Focused inspection

Look for asymmetry, nipple changes, scars, skin changes, skin tethering, *peau d'orange*, lumps and swellings, effects of radiotherapy, and lymphoedema.

- 'Slow arm abduction' (accentuates asymmetry)
- 'Hands behind head' (inspect axillae for scars, swellings, radiotherapy; inframammary folds – lift each breast)
- 'Hands on hips and press in' (tenses pectorals and accentuates asymmetry, deep structure tethering, and absence in radical mastectomy)
- 'Forward lean' (accentuates abnormalities in large pendulous breasts)
- Inspect the back (evidence of latissimus dorsi reconstruction)
- Inspect the abdomen (evidence of TRAM flap reconstruction)
- Surgical sequelae after mastectomy:
  - sensation in the armpit and lateral chest wall (intercostobrachial nerve; T2)
  - scapula winging (long thoracic nerve of Bell; C5, C6, C7).

→ Palpation

Examine both breasts, beginning with the unaffected side (redress other breast to preserve dignity).

- 'Any tenderness?'
- 'Hand behind head and tilt to contralateral side' (breast then lies flat on chest wall).
- Palpate seven areas in each breast for lumps (four quadrants; axillary tail of Spence; nipple-areolar complex; inframammary fold).
- In clinical practice you should also palpate the retro-areolar tissue to try to express nipple discharge (but unlikely to be required in the MRCS OSCE).
- Palpate in the axilla for lymph nodes (four walls and apex).
- Inspect the supraclavicular lymph nodes.

Discovered lump

- 'Press hands into hips' for pectoralis contraction and palpate for fixity and tethering.
- Define lump characteristics.

→ Further considerations

- Physical examination of the chest (lungs), back, abdomen (hepatomegaly), neurological system (brain metastasis).
- Assess fitness for surgery.

→ Thank the patient and wash your hands

→ Summarise and offer your differential diagnosis

→ Introduction

- Introduce yourself to the patient.
- Ask for a nurse chaperone.
- Obtain consent.
- Ensure adequate privacy, patient comfort and exposure (position at 45°).
- Ask the patient whether they have any pain.
- Wash hands.

→ Inspection

Inspect from the foot of the bed and the patient's right-hand side.

General and peripheral stigmata

- Oxygen and ventilation adjuncts; ECG monitor; pulse oximeter.
- Look for anaemia and cyanosis (cardiorespiratory disease); tar stains; splinter haemorrhages (infective endocarditis); amputations (peripheral vascular disease); venous graft harvesting scars (long saphenous vein, radial artery).

Focused inspection

Look for chest scars (midline sternotomy, drains, pacemaker, implanted defibrillator); chest wall movements (asymmetry – respiratory dysfunction).

→ Palpation

- Warmth, pulse
- Sternotomy scar (malunion)
- Thrills
- Apex beat
- Other scars (pacemaker, defibrillator – usually left lateral infraclavicular area).

→ Auscultation

- Listen for apex beat, left lower sternal edge, left and right parasternal edge at 2nd intercostal spaces (murmurs, mechanical valves).
- Lung bases (heart failure).

→ Further considerations

- Physical examination of the respiratory system (lungs), peripheral vascular system (PVD) and abdomen (aortic aneurysm).
- Observation chart (HR, BP, temperature, RR, oxygen saturation).
- Urine dipstick (haematuria – infective endocarditis).
- ECG and chest X-ray.

You palpate an enlarged spleen. What might be causing it?

- Infection:
  - virus (EBV, CMV, HIV)
  - bacteria (typhoid, typhus, TB, sepsis, bacterial endocarditis)
  - protozoa (malaria, schistosomiasis, kala-azar)
- Haematological:
  - benign (haemolytic anaemias, pernicious anaemia, idiopathic thrombocytopenic purpura, sickle cell disease)
  - malignant (myeloproliferative, lymphoproliferative disorders)
- Vascular: portal hypertension
- Metabolic: amyloidosis; rheumatoid arthritis (Felty's syndrome); Gaucher's; systemic lupus erythematosus (SLE); sarcoidosis
- Other: cysts.

What might cause both the liver and spleen to be enlarged?

- Portal hypertension
- Myeloproliferative disorders
- Lymphoproliferative disorders.

Chronic liver disease: example

What are the classical stigmata of chronic liver disease?
Hands

- Leuconychia (hypoalbuminaemia)
- Clubbing
- Palmar erythema
- Dupuytren's contracture
- Bruising (coagulopathy)
- Liver flap (encephalopathy)
- Pruritus/scratch marks (accumulation of bile salts in the skin).

Face

- Jaundice (hyperbilirubinaemia)
- Scratch marks
- Spider naevi (portal hypertension)
- Foetor hepaticus.

Chest

- Gynaecomastia (oestrogen metabolism dysfunction)
- Loss of body hair
- Spider naevi (portal hypertension)
- Bruising
- Pectoral muscle wasting.

Abdomen
■ Signs of portal hypertension (hepatosplenomegaly, ascites, caput medusae)
■ Testicular atrophy.

Legs
■ Oedema (hypoalbuminaemia)
■ Muscle wasting
■ Bruising.

Stoma: examination

Common stomas include ileostomy, colostomy, ileal conduit, nephrostomy, urostomy and tracheostomy.

→ ## Introduction

■ Introduce yourself to the patient.
■ Ask for a nurse chaperone.
■ Obtain consent.
■ Ensure adequate privacy, patient comfort and exposure (lie flat with one pillow).
■ Ask the patient whether they have any pain.
■ Wash hands.

→ ## Inspection

Inspect from the foot of the bed and the patient's right-hand side.
■ Site: quadrant; well sited away from bony prominences, scars, skin folds?
■ Scars: previous surgery and stomas
■ Contents: liquid faeces; formed faeces; urine
■ Morphology: spout (ileostomy) or flush (colostomy)
■ Lumen: single (end stoma) or double (loop stoma)
■ Loop stoma:
  • presence of a bridge (a newly formed stoma)
  • identify afferent limb (produces stool output and is usually larger and more caudally placed to prevent spillover into efferent limb)
  • identify efferent limb (allows passage of flatus and mucous discharge from defunctioned distal bowel and is usually smaller and more cephalically placed)
■ State of the stoma: ischaemia/necrosis; ulceration; stenosis
■ Surrounding skin: excoriation and erythema (? poorly fitting bag)
■ Parastomal hernia (lift head off bed and cough)
■ Prolapse or retraction
■ Mucocutaneous separation
■ Output: high (e.g. in ileostomy).

→ Palpation

- Digital stomal exam: insert a finger into the stoma to check stoma patency and for stenosis (and ensure bag is re-applied)
- Illuminate stomal tract: shine a light into the stoma to check the integrity of the mucosa.

→ Further considerations

- Inspection of perineum for scars and presence of anal opening
- Complete examination of abdomen
- Assess stoma postion during sitting, lying and standing.

→ Thank the patient and wash your hands

→ Summarise and offer your differential diagnosis

Groin: examination

→ Introduction

- Introduce yourself to the patient.
- Ask for a nurse chaperone.
- Obtain consent.
- Ensure adequate privacy, patient comfort and exposure. Stand the patient up and obtain full exposure of the groin, genitalia and abdomen. However, be prepared to be flexible depending on the patient's mobility.
- Ask the patient whether they have any pain.
- Wash hands.

Each time you ask the patient to cough, there should be a precise purpose. Examiners will be watching how many times you make the patient cough and at which stage.

→ Inspection

- Lump in the groin: define its characteristics
- Scars (especially overlying any lumps)
- *Cough 1*: look away and cough (inspect superficial ring of affected side for a cough impulse)
- *Cough 2*: look away and cough (inspect superficial ring of contralateral side).

→ Palpation

Stand to the patient's side with one hand on their back and the other hand on the lump itself.

- Any pain?

■ Can you get above the lump? If you cannot, it is likely to be a groin swelling and you should proceed as below. If you can get above the lump, it is likely to be a scrotal lump
■ Site:
  • key landmarks (anterior superior iliac spine, pubic tubercle, the interposed inguinal ligament, femoral artery pulsation)
  • relations to pubic tubercle (femoral versus inguinal hernia)
■ Lump characteristics
■ *Cough 3*: expansile cough impulse
■ Reducibility: ask patient 'to push it back in if possible' (direct course – direct hernia; oblique course – indirect hernia)
■ *Cough 4*: place one finger on pubic tubercle and ask the patient to cough again (note the relation of lump to the pubic tubercle as it protrudes):
  • *above and medial to the pubic tubercle* = inguinal hernia
  • *below and lateral to the pubic tubercle* = femoral hernia
■ *Cough 5* (deep ring occlusion test):
  • Place one hand on the deep inguinal ring, above a point half way between the pubic tubercle and the anterior superior iliac spine, and then ask the patient to look away and cough. If the lump is controlled then the inguinal hernia is indirect.

→ Auscultation

Listen for bowel sounds to assess viability of the bowel.

→ Further considerations

■ Examination of contralateral groin
■ Examination of genitalia for coincidental hydrocele or varicocele
■ Examination of regional lymph nodes
■ Full history
■ Examination of the abdomen
■ Digital rectal examination
■ Assess fitness for surgery.

You have found a lump in the groin. What do you think it is?

This is best tackled anatomically with pathologies related to each layer. The differentials include:
■ Skin – sebaceous cyst
■ Subcutaneous tissues – lipoma, fibroma
■ Lymphatics – inguinal lymphadenopathy
■ Bowel – inguinal or femoral hernia
■ Vein – saphena varix
■ Artery – femoral artery aneurysm
■ Nerve – neuroma or neurofibroma
■ Spermatic cord – lipoma of the cord; encysted hydrocele of cord

- Testis/scrotum – ectopic testis
- Muscle – benign or malignant tumour
- Psoas sheath – psoas abscess or psoas bursa.

→ Thank the patient and wash your hands

→ Summarise and offer your differential diagnosis

External male genitalia: examination

→ Introduction

- Introduce yourself to the patient.
- Ask for a nurse chaperone.
- Obtain consent.
- Ensure adequate privacy, patient comfort and exposure. Stand the patient up and obtain full exposure of the groin, genitalia and abdomen. However, be prepared to be flexible depending on the patient's mobility.
- Ask the patient whether they have any pain.
- Wash hands.

→ Inspection

- Lumps in the groin: look away and cough.
- Scars (including posterior aspect of scrotum).

→ Palpation

- Any pain?
- Can you get above the lump? If you can get above the lump, it is likely to be a scrotal lump and you should proceed as below. If you cannot, it is likely to be a groin swelling
- Relations to testis: assess whether the lump is separable from the testis
- Lump characteristics
- Relations to scrotal skin and scrotal skin pathology
- Transillumination: bright (hydrocele, epididymal cyst)
- Cough impulse: look away and cough (indirect hernia).

Examine the contralateral side, and examine the patient in the standing position to avoid missing a varicocele.

→ Further considerations

- Full history
- Examination of the abdomen
- Digital rectal examination
- Assess fitness for surgery.

→ Thank the patient and wash your hands

→ Summarise and offer your differential diagnosis

Model for an orthopaedic history

B&L **For further reading see *Bailey and Love*, Chapter 31.**

→ ## Introduction

Set the stage
- Welcome the patient, and ensure comfort and privacy.
- Know and use the patient's name.
- Introduce and identify yourself.

Set the agenda
- Begin with open-ended questions to ascertain the patient's perspective.
- Encourage the consultations with silences, and non-verbal and verbal cues.
- Focus by paraphrasing and summarising.

→ ## Personal information

Name; age; occupation; ethnic origin.

→ ## Presenting complaint in the patient's own words

→ ## History of presenting complaint

- System-specific:
  - muscle, bone or joint pain (location, time, mode of onset, severity, nature, progression, quantity, quality, frequency, duration, relieving and exacerbating factors, associated symptoms, radiation)
  - deformity
  - swelling
  - stiffness
  - limb weakness
  - reduced range of movement
  - effects on function
- Risk factors
- Investigations and treatment.

→ ## Past medical, surgical and anaesthetic history

→ ## Medication, allergies and immunisations

→ Family history

→ Social history

- Marital status
- Occupation and exposures
- Smoking history
- Alcohol consumption
- Illicit drug use
- Living accommodation
- Recent travel history.

→ Systems review

- General/constitutional
- Skin/breast
- Eyes/ears/nose/mouth/throat
- Cardiovascular
- Respiratory
- Gastrointestinal
- Genitourinary
- Musculoskeletal
- Neurological
- Psychiatric
- Immunologic/lymphatic/endocrine.

→ Thank the patient and wash your hands

→ Summarise and offer your differential diagnosis

Hip joint: examination

→ Introduction

- Start with the patient standing with a fully exposed hip joint.
- Ask the patient whether they have any pain.
- Wash hands.
- Examination of the hip (ball and socket) joint follows the same logical pattern as examination of any other joint. This includes:
  - look
  - feel
  - move
  - special tests.

→ Look

General

■ Look around the bed for walking aids and shoe-raises.
■ Look at the patient as a whole: well/unwell; pain/pain-free.
■ Assess gait, noting an antalgic or Trendelenburg gait.
■ Assess posture.
■ Assess for leg length inequality – true (due to a short leg) or apparent (result of a hip deformity) (see below).

Specific

■ Inspect for swelling, muscle wasting, signs of inflammation and sinus formation.
■ *Anterior*: scars; wasting of quadriceps; sinuses; fixed flexion deformity or rotational deformities. Put your hands on both anterior superior iliac fossae (ASIS) to check whether they are level (assess for pelvic tilt).
■ *Lateral*: scars; wasting muscles; sinuses and exaggerated lordosis of the spine.
■ *Posterior*: scars; wasting glutei/hamstrings; tufts of hair; scoliosis; sinuses.

→ Feel

Ask the patient whether they are in pain before you begin.

■ Assess the temperature of the joint with the back of your hand.
■ Palpate for local tenderness over this ball and socket joint and soft tissues.
■ The hip joint lies posterior to the femoral artery at the mid-inguinal point (half way between the ASIS and the symphysis pubis).
■ Palpate the ischial tuberosity, greater trochanter, and tendon of adductor longus.
■ Assess for inguinal lymph nodes.

→ Move

See Fig. 6.4.1.

■ Assess for joint crepitus, while moving the hip joint (with one hand over the hip joint, roll the femur laterally and medially).
■ Perform Thomas' test. This assesses for a fixed flexion deformity (FFD) of the hip joint. While the patient is in a supine position, place your hand between the patient's lumbar supine and the examination couch. Obliterate the lumbar lordosis by flexing the patient's good hip (ask the patient to bring their knee up towards their chest and hold it). This should compress your hand between their lumbar spine and the couch. The opposite leg should remain flat on the couch. Now you may exclude an FFD of the bad hip. The opposite leg will lift off the couch demonstrating the amount of flexion deformity present.

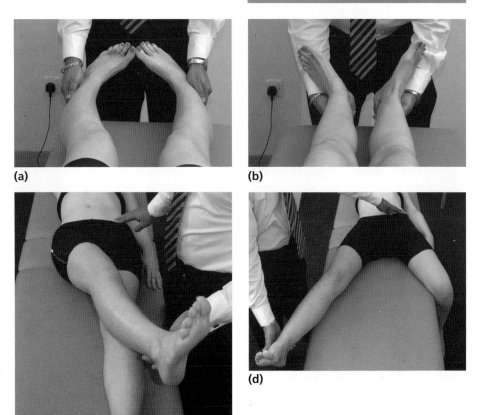

(a)

(b)

(c)

(d)

Figure 6.4.1 ● Hip movements: (a) internal rotation; (b) external rotation; (c) adduction; (d) abduction. (Bailey and Love, Figures 31.26a–31.26d, p.445.)

- Hip flexion has already been assessed in Thomas' test. The normal range of hip flexion is 0–120°.
- Test for abduction/adduction of the hip, while immobilising the pelvis by placing your hand on the contralateral ASIS to fix the pelvis. Then abduct (45°) and adduct (25°) each hip. Assess the range of movement and note any crepitus.
- Test for internal and external rotation (in extension) by looking at the patellae (90° arc of movement). Assess the range of movement and note any crepitus.
- Test internal (30°) and external (45°) rotation with the hip flexed (flex the hip and knee to 90°). Assess the range of movement and note any crepitus.

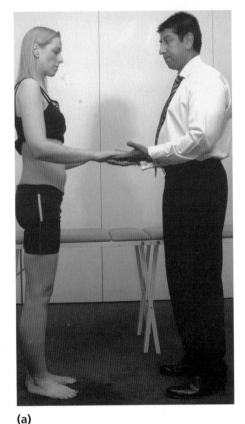

(a)

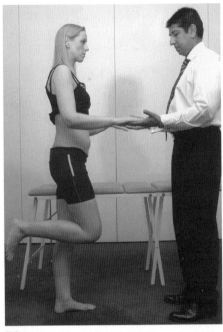

(b)

Figure 6.4.2 ● Trendelenburg test. (Bailey and Love, Figures 31.28a and 31.28b, p.446.)

→ ## Special tests

Trendelenburg's test

Face the standing patient (Fig. 6.4.2). Have the patient rest their hands on your shoulders or on your hands. This will support the patient and prevent them from falling over. Put your hands on their anterior superior iliac spines or look at their hips, to assess for a pelvic tilt. First, ask the patient to stand on their good leg while flexing the non-weight-bearing leg at the knee to 90°. Then repeat the test on the other leg. When a person stands on one leg, the glutei muscles contract so the opposite side of the pelvis is tilted up slightly to allow the leg to clear the ground on walking.

Positive Trendelenburg sign: If the actions of the glutei muscles are deficient, the opposite side of the pelvis will tilt downwards and the patient maintains balances by leaning over towards the side of the problem.

Assessing leg lengths

The patient should be in a supine position. Square the pelvis and place the legs in comparable positions. A fixed flexion deformity of the hip joint is present when the legs are unequal in length when they are in a parallel position.

- *Apparent leg length* is measured between fixed points, for example from the xiphisternum or umbilicus to the tip of the malleolus.
- *True leg length* is measured from the anterior superior iliac spine (ASIS) to the medial malleolus.

The Galeazzi test is performed with the patient's heels together. Examine the patient from the side and the end of the examination couch. Assess whether the leg shortening originates from the femur (above knee) or the tibia (below knee). If you are unclear, flex the hip and knee joints to 90° and look at the knees from the side.

→ **Further considerations**

- Assess the neurovascular status of the lower limbs.
- Examine the joint above and below (spine/knee).
- Assess the impact of the joint condition on the patient's life.
- Request an X-ray of the hip joint.
- Assess the patient's fitness for surgery.

→ **Thank the patient and wash your hands**

→ **Summarise and offer your differential diagnosis**

Knee joint: examination

→ **Introduction**

- Start with the patient standing and fully expose the knee joint.
- Ask the patient whether they have any pain.
- Wash hands.
- Examination of the knee (hinge) joint follows the same logical pattern as examination of any other joint. This includes:
  - look
  - feel
  - move
  - special tests.

→ **Look**

General

- Look around the bed for walking aids, shoe-raises etc.
- Look at the patient as a whole: well/unwell; pain/pain-free.
- Ask the patient to walk and squat.

Specific

Patient standing:

- Inspect for swelling, muscle wasting, signs of inflammation and sinus formation.

■ *Anterior with the legs together*: scars; wasting of quadriceps muscle; sinuses; fixed flexion deformities and valgus/varus deformities (alignment).

■ *Lateral*: scars; wasting muscles; sinuses and fixed flexion deformity.

■ *Posterior*: scars; popliteal swellings.

Patient supine:

■ Inspect for effusion: look for a 'horseshoe' swelling of the suprapatellar pouch.

■ Inspect for scars, including arthroscopic scars either side of the patellar tendon, anteromedially and anterolaterally.

→ Feel

Ask the patient whether they are in pain before you begin.

■ Assess the temperature of the joint with the back of your hand.

■ If you noted quadriceps muscle wasting on inspection, now measure the leg circumference 15 cm above the tibial tubercle.

■ Ask the patient to push their heels down into the bed and feel the bulk of the quadriceps muscle. To exclude a fixed flexion deformity, place your hand behind the popliteal fossa. If an FFD is present, place one hand on the patella and one hand on the quadriceps muscle and straighten the knee joint, to confirm it is fixed.

■ Assess for a knee joint effusion:

• For small effusions, perform the 'swipe test' and inspect for loss of the medial sulcus.

• For moderate effusions, perform the 'patellar tap test'. With the knee extended, empty the suprapatellar pouch by pressure of your hand. With your other hand, press against the patella sharply against the femur to produce a 'tap'.

• For large effusions, ballot the fluid between the medial and lateral aspects of the joint ('cross fluctuation test').

■ Palpate for local tenderness over this hinge joint and soft tissues. Flex the patient's knee to 45° and palpate this joint systematically (medial tibial condyle, medial joint line, medial femoral condyle, medial collateral ligament, tibial tuberosity, posteriorly in the popliteal fossa, lateral femoral condyle, lateral joint line, lateral tibial condyle, lateral collateral ligament and head of the fibula).

■ Now straighten the knee joint and palpate the patella in two planes (assess for patellofemoral joint crepitus and tenderness).

■ Palpate along the extensor mechanism for gaps or defects.

■ Assess for popliteal lymph nodes.

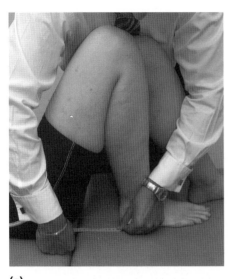

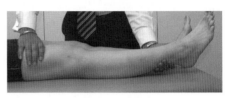

(b)

Figure 6.4.3 ● Knee flexion and extension. (Bailey and Love, Figures 31.29a and 31.29b, p.447.)

(a)

→ Move

- Place your hand on the knee joint to detect crepitus on movement and then ask the patient to flex the knee (bring the patient's heel to their bottom). The range of movement is 0–150°. At the limit of movement, assess the range of passive movement (Fig. 6.4.3).
- Inspect for an intact extension apparatus, flexion contractures and 'extensor lag' on straight leg raising. Ask the patient to point their toes to the ceiling, perform a straight leg raise and then return the leg to the examination couch.
- Assess for hyperextension (genu recurvatum) by placing your hand on the patient's patella and lift their heel upwards.

→ Special tests

Collateral ligaments
See Fig. 6.4.4.
- *Valgus/varus stress*: With the patient's knee fully extended, hold the patient's ankle in your axilla. With both of your hands, abduct and adduct the femur while keeping the patient's knee joint in extension and then in flexion.

Cruciate ligaments
- *Posterior sag test*: Place the patient's heels together, knees flexed to 45° and inspect from the side.
- *Drawer test*: With the patient's knees flexed to 45°, inform and then sit on or stabilise the patient's feet (Fig. 6.4.5). Excessive anterior draw is due to laxity of the anterior cruciate, and posterior sag is associated with laxity of the posterior cruciate ligament.

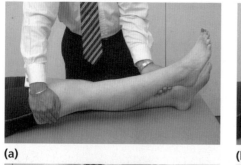

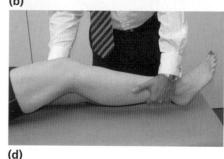

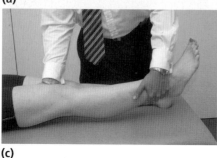

(a) **(b)**

(c) **(d)**

Figure 6.4.4 ● Assessing the medial and lateral collateral ligaments. (Bailey and Love, Figures 31.30a–31.30d, p.448.)

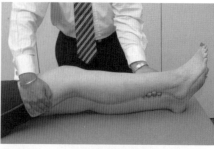

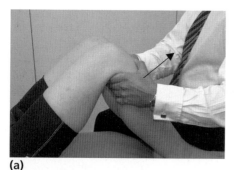

(a)

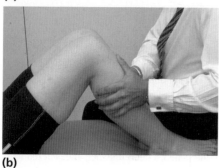

(b)

Figure 6.4.5 ● (a) Anterior draw test for anterior cruciate ligament stability. (b) Posterior draw test for posterior cruciate ligament stability. (Bailey and Love, Figures 31.32a and 31.32b, p.448.)

- *Lachman's test*: Flex the patient's knee to 15–30° (Fig. 6.4.6). Hold the lower end of the thigh in your one hand and the upper end of the tibia with the other. Push the lower thigh in one direction and pull the tibia in the opposite direction and then in the reverse directions.

Menisci

- *McMurray's test*: Flex and externally rotate the knee and then slowly extend the knee to stress the medial meniscus. Flex and internally rotate the knee and then slowly extend the knee to stress the lateral meniscus. Palpate for click and assess for focal tenderness during the test as it may suggest a tear.

Patella

- *Lateral apprehension test*: With the patient's knee in extension, apply pressure against the medial border of the patella. Maintain the pressure, while flexing the knee to 30° and assess the degree of patella movement. Inspect the patient's face for apprehension.

→ Further considerations

■ Assess the neurovascular status of the lower limbs.
■ Examine the joint above and below (spine/hip/ankle joints).
■ Assess the impact of the joint condition on the patient's life.
■ Request a weight-bearing X-ray of the knee joint.
■ Assess the patient's fitness for surgery.

→ Thank the patient and wash your hands

→ Summarise and offer your differential diagnosis

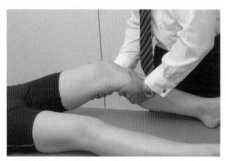

Figure 6.4.6 ● Lachman's test. Flex the knee to 15–30 degrees and pull the proximal tibia forwards. (Bailey and Love, Figure 31.31, p.448.)

Shoulder joint: examination

→ Introduction

■ Start with the patient standing and fully expose the shoulder joint.
■ Ask the patient whether they have any pain.
■ Wash hands.
■ Examination of the shoulder (ball and socket) joint follows the same logical pattern as examination of any other joint. This includes:
  • look
  • feel
  • move
  • special tests.

→ Look

General
■ Look around the bed for aids (slings).
■ Look at the patient as a whole: well/unwell; pain/pain-free.

Specific

Patient standing:

- Inspect for swelling, muscle wasting, signs of inflammation and sinus formation.
- *Anterior*: arthroscopic scars; sinuses; contour of the shoulder/squaring off; muscle wasting of deltoid and trapezius.
- *Lateral*: scars.
- *Posterior*: scars, contour and muscle wasting of supraspinatus/infraspinatus.
- Ask the patient to push with their hands against a wall. Inspect for winging of the scapula (serratus anterior muscle supplied by long thoracic nerve of Bell, C5/6/7).

→ ## Feel

Ask the patient whether they are in pain before you begin.

- Assess the temperature of the joint with the back of your hand.
- Palpate over the sternoclavicular joint, along the clavicle, coracoid process, acromion/acromioclavicular joint, subacromial space, abduct the humerus and then palpate the glenohumeral joint line into the axilla. Continue posteriorly to assess the greater tuberosity of humerus, spine of scapula, inferior pole of scapula, supraspinatus and infraspinatus.
- Assess for axillary lymph nodes.

→ ## Move

See Fig. 6.4.7.

- Place your hand on the shoulder joint to detect crepitus on passive movement.
- *Forward flexion*: With the patient's arm by the side, ask the patient to flex the shoulder forward (90°) (Fig. 6.4.7a).
- *Extension* (Fig. 6.4.7b).
- *Abduction*: Ask the patient to abduct the arm (90°). Assess for a 'painful arc' (Fig. 6.4.8).
- *Adduction*: Ask the patient to bring their arm over to the opposite shoulder (assess for osteoarthritis of the acromioclavicular joint at this point = Scarf test) (Fig. 6.4.7c).
- *Internal rotation*: Ask the patient to place their hands behind their back (normally one should be able to reach up as high as the 6th thoracic vertebrae) (Fig. 6.4.7d).
- *External rotation*: Flex the patient's elbows to 90° and then ask the patient to place their hands behind their head (Fig. 6.4.7e).

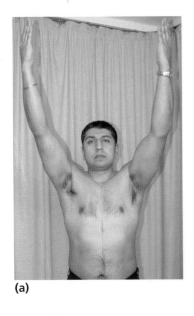

(a)

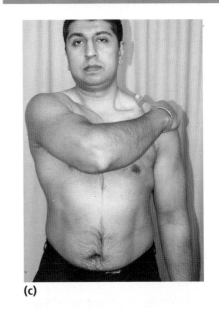

(c)

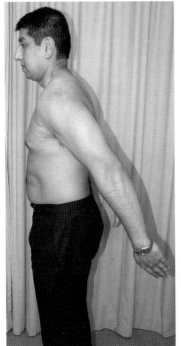

(b)

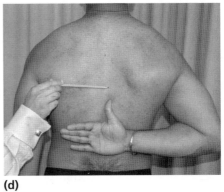

(d)

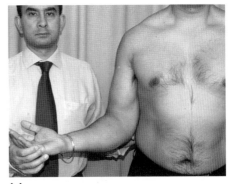

(e)

Figure 6.4.7 ● Movements of the shoulder: (a) forward flexion; (b) extension; (c) adduction; (d) internal rotation; (e) external rotation. (Bailey and Love, Figures 31.22a–31.22e, p.442.)

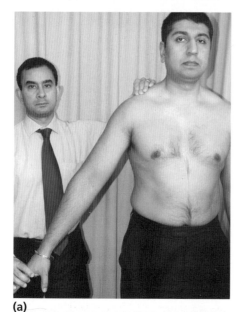

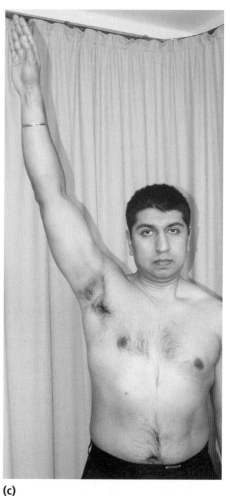

(a)

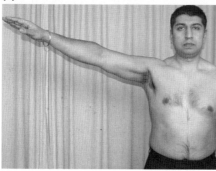

(b)

(c)

Figure 6.4.8 ● Painful arc test for rotator cuff impingement. (Bailey and Love, Figures 31.23a–31.23c, p.443.)

→ Special tests

Rotator cuff muscles

- *Supraspinatus* (thumbs down test/Jobe's test/empty-can test): Ask the patient to abduct their arm against resistance (Fig. 6.4.9). To exclude rupture, passively abduct the patient's arm to 40°, then the patient should be able to continue active abduction.
- *Teres minor and infraspinatus*: resisted external rotation.
- *Subscapularis*: Gerber's lift-off test.

Impingement test

- *Hawkin's test*: Raise the patient's arm to 90° forward flexion and bend the elbow to 90° (Fig. 6.4.10). Then passively internally rotate the shoulder (i.e. thumb pointed down). Pain is indicative of impingement.

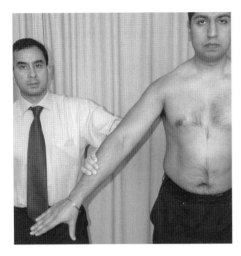

Figure 6.4.9 ● Jobe's test for rotator cuff impingement. (Bailey and Love, Figure 31.24, p.444.)

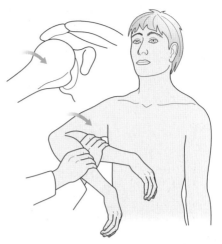

Figure 6.4.10 ● Hawkin's impingement test. Impingement pain is reproduced when the shoulder is internally rotated with 90 degrees of forward flexion, thereby locating the greater tuberosity underneath the acromion. (Bailey and Love, Figure 34.5, p.487.)

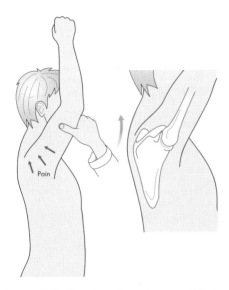

Figure 6.4.11 ● Neer's impingement test. Pain is reproduced with full forward flexion. (Bailey and Love, Figure 34.6, p.487.)

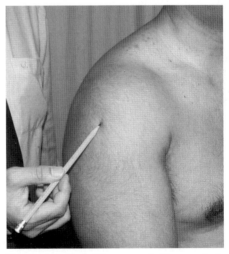

Figure 6.4.12 ● The area of skin supplied by the axilliary nerve: 'the regimental badge area'. (Bailey and Love, Figure 31.21, p.441.)

■ *Neer's sign and test*: With the patient's thumb down, place your hand on their shoulder and with your other hand passively lift up their hand in the plane of the scapula (forward flexion) until they express pain (Fig. 6.4.11). Pain during this manoeuvre is a positive Neer's sign, and pain abolished with local anaesthetic is a positive Neer's test.

Ruptured head of biceps
- Assess for a 'biceps bulge' on flexing the patient's elbow against resistance.

Axillary nerve function
- Assess for deltoid muscle power and sensation (fine touch) in the regimental badge area (Fig. 6.4.12).

→ ## Further considerations
- Assess the neurovascular status of the upper limbs.
- Examine the joint above and below (cervical spine and elbow joint).
- Assess the impact of the joint condition on the patient's life.
- Request X-rays (including axillary view) of the shoulder joint.
- Assess the patient's fitness for surgery.

→ ## Thank the patient and wash your hands

→ ## Summarise and offer your differential diagnosis

Spine: examination

→ ## Introduction
- Start with the patient standing and fully exposed.
- Ask the patient whether they have any pain.
- Wash hands.
- Examination of the spine follows the same logical pattern as examination of any other joint. This includes:
  - look
  - feel
  - move
  - special tests.

→ ## Look

General
- Look around the bed for walking aids and supports (Miami J collar, thoracolumbar brace).
- Look at the patient as a whole: well/unwell; pain/pain-free.
- Ask the patient to walk in order to assess gait.
- Ask the patient to stand on their heels (L4/L5) and toes (S1/S2).

Specific
Patient standing:
- Skin: scars; sinuses; hairy tufts; café au lait spots
- Soft tissues: muscle wasting
- Bone: scoliosis, kyphosis, lumbar lordosis, gibbus.

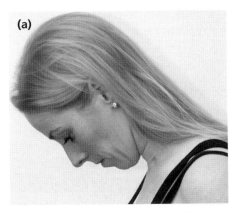
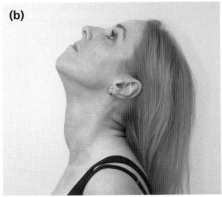
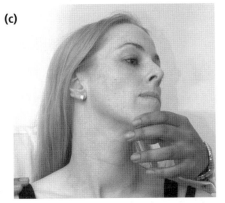
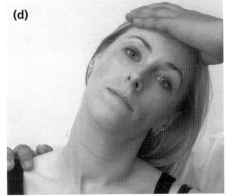

Figure 6.4.13 ● Cervical spine (a,b) flexion/
extension, (c) rotation, and (d) bending.
(Bailey and Love, Figures 31.3a–31.3d, p.433.)

→ Feel

Ask the patient whether they are in pain before you begin.
- Assess the temperature of the spine with the back of your hand.
- Palpate and percuss over the entire spine for any bony or muscle tenderness, and assess for step deformities.

→ Move

Cervical spine

See Fig. 6.4.13.
- Ask the patient to move the head forward and backwards (flexion 75° and extension 60°).
- Ask the patient to look to the right and left (80° each direction).
- Ask the patient to tilt their head to the right and left towards their ear (lateral flexion 45° each direction).

Thoracic spine

- Ask the patient to rotate while sitting.
- Measure chest expansion.

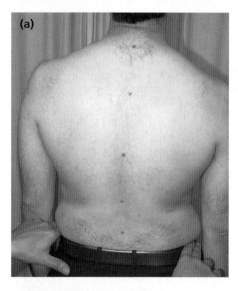

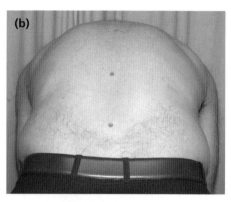

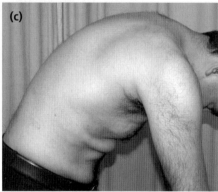

Figure 6.4.14 ● Forward bending test. (Bailey and Love, Figures 31.5a–31.5c, p.433.)

Lumbar spine

- *Forward flexion*: Ask the patient to touch their toes (if limited, perform Schober's test). The patient should be able to reach within 7 cm of the floor (Fig. 6.4.14).
- *Extension*: Ask the patient to bend backward (30°).
- *Lateral flexion*: Ask the patient to slide their hand down one side of the body (30°).
- *Rotation*: Ask the patient to sit down, cross their hands across their body and rotate their body (40°).

→ ## Special tests

Cervical spine

- *Lhermitte's sign* (the barber's chair phenomenon): This is demonstrated when you ask the patient to bend their cervical neck forward. This produces a radicular pain down the spine and into the upper limb. A positive test represents cervical nerve root compression.

Lumbar spine

- *Straight leg raise and sciatic nerve test*: Examine the patient in a supine position. With the patient's knee flexed, first check that passive hip flexion is normal. With the patient's knees extended, raise the patient's leg while supporting the patient's heel. On the affected side, the patient will experience pain at a certain level. At this limit, gently dorsiflex the ankle, which will apply further tension on the nerve root (Bragard's sign). Ensure you measure the angle the leg is elevated off the examination couch.
- *Femoral stretch test*: Ask the patient to lie prone. Flex the patient's knee and ask the patient to inform you when they have pain. The test is positive if the patient has pain radiating into their back.
- *Modified Schober's test*: Mark the level between the iliac crests and 10 cm above. Ask the patient to touch their toes. There should be more than 5 cm increase in separation.
- *Heel–hips–occiput test*: Also known as the 'wall test' (ankylosing spondylitis).
- *Patrick's test for sacro-iliac joint* (also known as the Faber test) and other SIJ tests.

→ **Further considerations**

- Full neurological assessment of the upper and lower limbs.
- Full vascular examination of the upper and lower limbs.
- Abdominal examination (to exclude an abdominal aortic aneurysm) and assess anal tone by performing a digital rectal examination.
- Examine the joint above and below (shoulder and hip joint).
- Assess the impact of the joint condition on the patient's life.
- X-rays of the spine (further imaging, including CT and MRI scans, should be considered.
- Assess the patient's fitness for surgery.

→ **Thank the patient and wash your hands**

→ **Summarise and offer your differential diagnosis**

Hand: examination

The hand examination may represent a rheumatologic, orthopaedic, neurological or vascular case. This section will focus on the 'rheumatoid hand' examination.

→ **Introduction**

- Start with the patient sitting. The patient's upper limbs should be fully exposed and their hands resting on a pillow.
- Ask the patient whether they have any pain.

- Wash hands.
- Examination of the hands follows the same logical pattern as examination of any other joint. This includes:
  - look
  - feel
  - move
  - special tests.

→ ## Look

General
- Look around the bed for aids and supports.
- Look at the patient as a whole: well/unwell; pain/pain-free.
- Ensure you assess for extra-articular manifestations of systemic disease (see below).

Specific: dorsal aspect of the patient's hands
- Skin and soft tissue:
  - nail changes (nail fold infarcts, pitting, vasculitic lesions, pale beds)
  - ulcers
  - rashes
  - bruising, purpura, and thinning of the skin (secondary to steroids)
  - swelling.
- Muscles:
  - wasting of intrinsic muscles (accentuates the extensor tendons)
  - dorsal guttering.
- Bones:
  - loss of the normal finger cascade
  - spindling of fingers
  - sparing of distal interphalangeal joints
  - ulnar deviation of fingers
  - Swan-neck deformity (hyperextended proximal interphalangeal joint but flexed distal joint) (Fig. 6.4.15)
  - Boutonnière deformity (flexed proximal interphalangeal joint, extended metacarpophalangeal joint, hyperextended distal interphalangeal joint)
    - metacarpophalangeal joints and wrist subluxation
    - radial deviation and volar subluxation at the wrist joint
    - z-deformities of the thumbs.

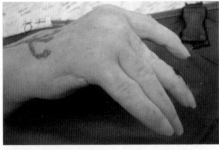

Figure 6.4.15 ● Swan-neck deformity.
(Bailey and Love, Figure 37.2, p.540.)

Specific: palmar/volar aspect of the patient's hands

Ask the patient to lift their hands off the pillow in order to expose the palmar aspects of the hands. Assess for a dropped finger/thumb (evidence of extensor tendon rupture) and wrist drop. Moreover, assess for range of movement (supination/pronation).

- Skin and deep fascia:
  - scars (carpal tunnel decompression; a dorsal wrist scar implies previous synovectomy or arthrodesis in rheumatoid arthritis; a scar over the head of the ulna implies a previous Darrach procedure)
  - pale palmar creases
  - palmar erythema
- Muscles: wasting of the thenar and hypothenar eminences
- Bones: fingers held in flexion
- Elbows: ask the patient to put their hands behind their head and check for:
  - scars around the medial epicondyle (ulnar nerve decompression)
  - rheumatoid nodules.

→ Feel

Ask the patient whether they are in pain before you begin.

- Assess the temperature of the hands with the back of your hand.
- Assess capillary refill time and ulnar and radial pulses.
- Squeeze the metacarpals together and assess for tenderness.
- Palpate each joint to ascertain the levels affected in the hand and whether active inflammation or inactive disease is present.
- Palpate for rheumatoid nodules (i.e. on pressure areas and tendon sheaths).
- Palpate for tendon ruptures (start your palpation on the ulnar side of the hands).

→ Move

Assess for active and passive movement at the wrist and fingers by asking the patient to perform the following movements:

- Grip and squeeze two of your fingers and perform a fine pinch.
- Flex one finger at a time while touching the thenar eminence.
- Spread fingers wide apart.
- Demonstrate playing the piano with the fingers.
- Oppose thumb to each finger.
- Place their hands in a 'praying position' to demonstrate wrist dorsiflexion.
- Place their hands in a 'reverse praying position' to demonstrate wrist flexion.

→ ## Special tests

Functional assessment
- Power grip
- Pincer grip (pick up a coin or key)
- Button and unbutton shirt
- Hold a pen and write.

Neurological assessment (sensation)
- Radial nerve (dorsum of first interosseous web-space)
- Median nerve (palmar/volar aspect of index finger)
- Ulnar nerves (palmar/volar aspect of little finger).

Table top test
- Ask the patient to place their hands flat on a table.

→ ## Further considerations

- Full neurological assessment of the upper limbs.
- Full vascular examination of the upper limbs.
- Examine the joint above (wrist and elbow joints).
- Assess other joint involvement (hip, knee, shoulder, spine).
- Assess for extra-articular manifestations of rheumatoid disease: see Table 6.4.1.

Table 6.4.1
Extra-articular manifestations of rheumatoid disease

Location	Effects
Systemic	Weight loss; fever; malaise; vasculitis; amyloidosis
Skin	Subcutaneous (rheumatoid) nodules
Eyes	Keratoconjunctivitis sicca; scleritis; episcleritis
Cardiovascular	Pericardial effusion; pericarditis; myocarditis
Respiratory	Pleurisy; pleural effusion; nodules; fibrosing alveolitis
Neurological	Entrapment neuropathy (carpal tunnel syndrome); atlantoaxial instability; multifocal neuropathies
Abdominal	Splenomegaly, Felty's syndrome
Haematological	Anaemia; leucopenia; lymphadenopathy
Musculoskeletal	Knees (valgus/varus deformity, popliteal 'Baker's' cysts); scars for shoulder; knee or hip replacements

- Assess the impact of the joint condition on the patient's life.
- Request X-rays of the wrist and hand.
- Assess the patient's fitness for surgery.

→ ## Thank the patient and wash your hands

→ ## Summarise and offer your differential diagnosis

Model for a vascular history

→ Introduction

- Set the stage:
  - Welcome the patient and ensure comfort and privacy.
  - Introduce and identify yourself.
  - Know and use the patient's name.
- Set the agenda:
  - Begin with open-ended questions to ascertain the patient's perspective.
  - Encourage the consultations with silences and non-verbal and verbal cues.
  - Focus by paraphrasing and summarising.

→ Personal information

Name, age, occupation and ethnic origin.

→ Presenting complaint in the patient's own words

→ History of presenting complaint

System-specific: cardiac

- Angina: location; time; mode of onset; severity; nature; progression; quantity; quality; frequency; duration; relieving and exacerbating factors; associated symptoms; radiation
- Dyspnoea, including paroxysmal nocturnal, at rest and effort
- Orthopnoea
- Palpitations
- Headaches and dizziness
- Oedema (pulmonary, peripheral).

System-specific: peripheral vascular

- Limb pain: location; time; mode of onset; severity; nature; progression; quantity; quality; frequency; duration; relieving and exacerbating factors; associated symptoms; radiation
- Deformity
- Swelling
- Stiffness
- Amputations and ulceration
- Limb neurology: weakness; paraesthesia
- Reduced range of movement
- Effects on function
- Walking distance.

Risk factors: smoking; hypertension; diabetes; hypercholesterolaemia; family history of atherosclerosis; diet

Investigations and treatment (medical, endovascular and surgical)

→ Past medical, surgical and anaesthetic history

→ Medication, allergies and immunisations

→ Family history

Social history
- Marital status
- Occupation and exposures
- Smoking history
- Alcohol consumption
- Diet
- Illicit drug use
- Living accommodation
- Recent travel history.

System review
- General/constitutional
- Skin/breast
- Eyes/ears/nose/mouth/throat
- Respiratory
- Gastrointestinal
- Genitourinary
- Musculoskeletal
- Neurological
- Psychiatric
- Immunologic/lymphatic/endocrine.

→ Thank the patient and wash your hands

→ Summarise and offer your differential diagnosis

Peripheral vascular system (upper and lower limbs): examination

→ Introduction
- Start the examination with the patient supine with a pillow under their head for support. The patient's limbs (upper and lower) and chest should be fully exposed.
- Ask the patient whether they have any pain.
- Wash hands.

→ Inspection

General

- Look around the bed for aids, oxygen or medication (GTN spray).
- Look at the patient as a whole: well/unwell; pain/pain-free; shortness of breath; cyanosis; obesity.

Specific: upper limbs and trunk

- Skin and nails: tar staining; clubbing; brittle nails; splinter haemorrhages; vasculitic changes; pulp atrophy; digital colour changes/cyanosis; pale palmar creases; ulceration; gangrene; amputations

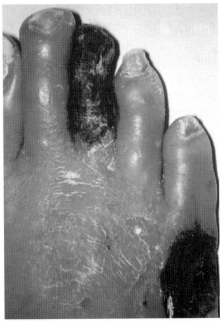

Figure 6.4.16 ● Severe chronic ischaemia with dry gangrene. (Bailey and Love, Figure 53.4, p.901.)

- Scars: arms; neck (endarterectomy); chest (midline sternotomy); axillae (axillobifemoral bypass grafts); abdomen (laparotomy for abdominal aortic aneurysm)
- Horner's syndrome
- Muscle wasting.

Specific: lower limbs

- Skin and nails: nail changes for friability; skin colour; ulceration; gangrene (Fig. 6.4.16); digital amputations/tissue loss; changes of coincidental venous disease; oedema (often due to dependency); hair loss; venous guttering
- Scars: vein harvest; reconstruction procedures; grafts/flaps for soft tissue cover of ulcers and areas of tissue loss; scars in the groin (exposure of common femoral artery)
- Muscles: wasting (often due to disuse atrophy); loss of prominence of extensor tendons on the dorsum of foot (oedema).
- Don't forget to examine between the toes.

→ Palpation

Ask the patient whether they are in pain before you begin.

Upper limbs

- Assess the temperature of the upper limbs with the back of your hand.
- Assess for the capillary refill time.
- Palpate the radial pulses for rate and rhythm. Moreover, assess for radial, radio-radial delay, collapsing pulse.
- Palpate the brachial pulse.
- Assess the patient's blood pressure in both upper limbs.
- Palpate the axillary artery in axilla.

- Palpate the subclavian artery (subclavian aneurysm, post-stenotic dilatation).
- Palpate the carotid pulses for rate, rhythm and character.
- Palpate the superficial temporal artery.
- Palpate for a cervical rib.

Lower limbs

- Assess the temperature of the lower limbs with the back of your hand.
- Assess for pitting oedema.
- Assess for capillary refill time.
- Palpate the abdomen for an abdominal aortic pulse.
- Palpate for a femoral pulse: midway between the ASIS and the symphysis pubis at the mid-inguinal point. Assess for a radio-femoral delay.
- Palpate for a popliteal pulse: flex the knee and wrap both hands around knee with fingertips into the popliteal fossa and compress artery against tibia posteriorly. Note the popliteal pulse is often difficult to assess as the popliteal artery lies deep within the popliteal fossa.
- Palpate the dorsalis pedis pulse: palpate between the head of the 1st and 2nd metatarsals. Ask the patient to bring their big toe towards their face. The pulse is lateral to the tendon of extensor hallucis longus. Note the dorsalis pedis pulse is absent in 10 per cent of normal individuals.
- Palpate the posterior tibial pulse: posterior to the medial malleolus.

→ ## Auscultation

Upper limbs

Listen for bruits in the supraclavicular fossa, infraclavicular space (subclavian) and over the carotid artery.

Lower limbs

Listen for bruits in the abdomen (aortic aneurysm, renal, iliacs), groin (femoral) and lower limb (adductor hiatus – lies two-thirds along a line drawn from the ASIS to the adductor tubercle).

→ ## Special tests

Ankle–brachial pressure index (ABPI)

Record the systolic blood pressure in the upper limbs and take the higher of the two readings. Locate the dorsalis pedis and posterior tibial pulses with the handheld Doppler (Fig 6.4.17) and inflate the cuff until the Doppler sound disappears. Slowly deflate and record the pressure at which the sound reappears. Take the higher of the two readings (posterior tibial or dorsalis pedis). The ABPI is the ratio of the best foot systolic to brachial systolic pressure (normal >1.0; claudication 0.4–0.7; critical ischaemia 0.1–0.4).

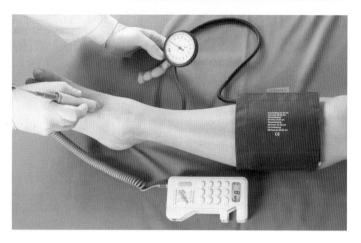

Figure 6.4.17 ● Handheld Doppler probe and sphygmomanometer used to determine systolic pressure in the dorsalis pedis artery, as part of assessing the ankle–brachial pressure index. (Bailey and Love, Figure 53.6, p.902.)

Allen's test

The patient should make a fist. Now occlude both radial and ulnar arteries. When the patient opens their palm, it should be white. You may now release the pressure on the ulnar artery (the hand should reperfuse). Repeat the test; i.e. make a fist, occlude both arteries, open palm, and now release the radial artery. This test demonstrates collateral circulation.

Buerger's test

Elevate the patient's straight leg off the examination couch. The leg angle from the examination couch when the leg turns white is Buerger's angle (<20° = severe ischaemia). Assist the patient in allowing them to drop their leg over the side of the couch and inspect for reactive hyperaemia.

→ Further considerations

- Full cardiovascular assessment.
- Full neurological examination of the upper and lower limbs.
- Full abdominal examination to exclude an abdominal aortic aneurysm.
- Exclude thoracic outlet obstruction (Adson's test, Wright's manoeuvre, and Roos' test).
- Use a handheld Doppler to assess pulses and character of waveforms, i.e. normal triphasic, biphasic (moderate stenosis), monophasic (severe stenosis), or absent waveforms.
- X-rays (CXR to identify a cervical rib) or CT scan (to identify an AAA).
- Arterial duplex.
- Arterial angiogram.
- Assess the impact of the condition on the patient's life.
- Assess the patient's fitness for surgery.

→ Thank the patient and wash your hands

→ Summarise and offer your differential diagnosis

Venous system: examination for varicose veins

→ ## Introduction

- Have the patient standing. The patient's groin and lower limbs should be fully exposed.
- Ask the patient whether they have any pain.
- Wash hands.

→ ## Inspection

General

- Look around the bed for walking aids and support stockings.
- Look at the patient as a whole: well/unwell; pain/pain-free.

Specific

- Ask the patient to stand with one leg in front of the other. You must inspect from the front, sides and behind.
- Assess for varicose veins (abnormal prominent superficial, tortuous and dilated veins) (Fig. 6.4.18). Note their distribution (long or short saphenous veins or both) and location (the medial gaiter area).
- Assess for surgical scars in the groin and lower limbs.
- Assess for saphena varix (varicosity in the saphenous vein at its confluence with the femoral vein).
- Inspect the lower limbs for 'chronic venous hypertension':
  - ulceration
  - haemosiderin deposition
  - thrombophlebitis
  - venous eczema and scars
  - lipodermatosclerosis ('inverted champagne bottle leg')
  - pitting oedema
  - healed ulceration (atrophie blanche) and ankle flare (corona phlebectatica)
  - loss of hair
  - shiny skin.

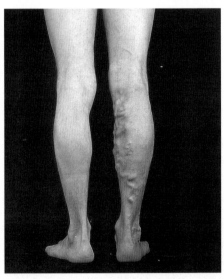

Figure 6.4.18 ● Varicose veins of the right leg. (Bailey and Love, Figure 54.3, p.927.)

→ ## Palpation

Ask the patient whether they are in pain before you begin.

- Assess the temperature of the lower limbs with the back of your hand.
- Assess for tenderness.
- Palpate the course of long and short saphenous veins.
- Palpate for pitting oedema.

- Palate the groin for regional lymph nodes.
- Palpate for a saphena varix.
- Perform the cough test to assess for a cough impulse or thrill. Identify the saphenofemoral junction (SFJ) in the groin (just medial to the femoral pulse). While your index finger is over this junction, ask the patient to cough.

→ Percussion

Perform the *tap test* (Chevrier's percussion test).
- Tap proximally and palpate distally (retrograde transmission) to detect venous valvular incompetence/reflux.
- Tap distally and palpate proximally (orthograde transmission) to assess venous continuity, venous patency and to detect thrombosis/venous occlusion.

→ Auscultation

Listen for bruits (arteriovenous fistulae).

→ Special tests

Tourniquet test
Also known as the Brodie-Trendelenburg test (if your fingers or thumb are placed over the SFJ, instead of using a tourniquet). Place the patient in a supine position, then elevate the lower limb to empty the veins. Apply a tourniquet high on the upper thigh and ask the patient to stand up. If the incompetence is above the tourniquet site, the veins will be controlled and will not fill. If the incompetence is below the level of the tourniquet, the vein will fill. This should be repeated with the tourniquet positioned at a lower level on the thigh.

Perthes' test
Place the tourniquet on the patient's thigh, Then ask the patient to stand on their toes. If the veins enlarge or the patient experiences pain, the deep veins are likely to be involved.

Handheld Doppler ultrasound
Doppler ultrasound is used to identify the femoral artery and the SFJ. Then compress the patient's calf. If there is venous incompetence at the SFJ, listen for backflow.

→ Further considerations

- ABPI of the lower limb.
- Venous duplex of the lower limbs.
- Full abdominal examination (pelvic exam, digital rectal exam and external genitalia) to exclude secondary causes of varicose veins.
- Assess the impact of the joint condition on the patient's life.
- Assess the patient's fitness for surgery.

Communication skills for the MRCS OSCE

The Communication Skills OSCE

Doctors must communicate effectively with patients, relatives, colleagues, and other professionals from an entire spectrum of socioeconomic and cultural backgrounds. This requires skills in verbal, non-verbal, written and telephone etiquette to quickly establish an appropriate and productive rapport to convey and receive information in a structured and comprehensive manner. Assessment of communication skills is a major feature of the MRCS OSCE and should not be underestimated. Although good communication skills are often second nature to caring, dynamic and articulate doctors, as with any exam there are effective techniques to maximise success.

Communication Skills OSCE stations are identical in length to the other stations (10 minutes) and may be manned or unmanned. The unmanned stations are usually written tasks such as writing a referral letter using a patient's medical notes. The manned stations generally begin with an opening minute for preparation of the clinical scenario with the information provided, followed by 9 minutes to act out the task. This could include discussion with a patient, relative, or another healthcare professional.

Communicating with a patient or relative
Typical scenarios include:
- taking a focused history
- breaking bad news
- explaining a procedure or obtaining consent
- dealing with angry or upset patients and relatives (complaints).

Communicating with another health professional
Typical scenarios include:
- writing a referral letter or discharge summary using clinical case notes
- making a direct referral face to face or over the phone.

It is clear that in order to complete these tasks effectively, adequate medical knowledge is essential. However, it is important to remember that it is the communication skills aspect that is being assessed primarily. With this in mind there are some useful framework models that can be applied to these stations, which always begin with meticulous systematic preparation.

Communication skills framework model

The Communication Skills OSCE is very much run by you, so you should have a structured, logical framework or game plan specific to this part of the exam. Here is a suggested format.

→ Preparation

- This involves the preparation time to work through the vignette, registering the task at hand and the salient information required from the material provided.
- You should map out the scenario including opening statements to the examiner, such as 'leaving your pager with a colleague to avoid being disturbed', 'selecting a private, tranquil room for the consultation'.
- You should rearrange the chairs to ensure that you are positioned in a non-defensive and approachable manner rather than across a desk. This demonstrates to the examiners that you have insight into social dynamics before you even begin the consultation.

→ Introductions

- First impressions are critical and can set the mood and fate for the remainder of the OSCE station.
- The patient, relative or colleague should be greeted by providing your name and position, as well as by inviting them to introduce themselves by name and affiliation to the patient (or position in the case of another healthcare professional).
- It is mandatory to state that you would ensure you have consent from the patient concerned if you are communicating with extended family members.
- The patient or relative should be asked whether they wish to be alone or accompanied by a friend, family member or nurse before proceeding any further.

→ Consultation

- This should commence with setting the scene and establishing what the patient, friend or other healthcare professional understands about the current medical condition.
- Use of appropriate verbal and non-verbal communication techniques is vital to avoid misunderstandings through miscommunication.
- Language should be pitched appropriately. Medical jargon may be justified when communicating with a colleague, but it is deemed inappropriate when communicating with a patient or relative.
- The sequence of open-ended questions, followed by direct questions, and then closed questions usually works well in most situations. This engages the person early on by empowering them in the conversation, building trust and a good rapport.
- Open questioning should address the person's **ideas, concerns** and **expectations** – 'ICE'. The nature of these obviously varies according to the person. For example, a patient may be hiding a plethora of psychosocial issues, whereas a busy intensivist might be trying to deal with the pressures of multiple teams fighting for that last ICU bed.

- Revealing the person's underlying agenda is often the key in the art of persuasion, as this then allows you to understand 'where they are coming from' and thus develop convincing arguments. For example, you might be consenting a patient for an operation whose close family member died on the operating table. Alternatively, you might be referring to the intensivist who will be waiting to hear clinical evidence that meets ICU admission criteria before accepting the referral.

- Body language and simple courtesy and etiquette are important aids to allow free flow of communication. Defensive positions (e.g. arms crossed and lack of eye contact) are often inhibitory to the consultation; whereas demonstrating an active interest – by repeating the salient points of what has been communicated and seeking clarification – tend to facilitate the process.

- Illustrations (pictures and diagrams) and patient information leaflets are helpful aids to demonstrate the important features of your discussion, which the patient or relative may take away with them. Other powerful tools include the use of silences and pauses to give the person space to think and express their true concerns.

- The power of smiling (if appropriate) cannot be underestimated as it removes intimidation and fear and introduces an air of calm and welcome. If, however, a patient or relative is upset and tearful, then empathy and compassion (and perhaps the offer of a tissue) may be appropriate.

- Use words the patient will understand (e.g. 'cancer') and avoid medical jargon (e.g. 'mitotic lesion', 'malignancy', 'growth') when breaking the bad news. Bear in mind that patients are often in a state of shock on hearing such loaded words and may not absorb any further information from that point onwards.

- Gauging a patient's non-verbal communication is often more pertinent than their verbal communication. In some cases it may be appropriate to continue the consultation another time.

- If a person is angry or aggressive, it is best to remain calm and ask them to explain their reasons so that you may understand their concerns. You should then reiterate what you have understood back to them and then offer a plan in an attempt to ameliorate the situation. Of course, if there has been a misunderstanding or mistake, you should offer an apology.

- It is important to stress that clinical knowledge is required to provide the medium through which communication skills are being assessed. However, in areas beyond your expertise it is correct and right to admit incomplete knowledge and state that you will consult a senior colleague or seek advice from experts in other disciplines (the multidisciplinary approach).

→ **Consolidation**

- You should ask the other person to repeat back what he or she has understood so far, which may then highlight whether there is any confusion or any further issues to address.
- If there is confusion, miscommunication or disagreement, these must be addressed at this time using 'ICE' once again, and then focusing in on the problem. This is obligatory when obtaining consent from a patient for a procedure.
- A patient has the right to refuse treatment if he or she has demonstrated an understanding of the facts.
- There may be times where an immediate solution or compromise cannot be reached. Scheduling a second meeting to discuss the matter further may well be the best option.

→ **Conclusion**

- You should summarise what has been communicated and provide an agreed management plan.
- Your name, position, and contact details should be given to the patient, relative or colleague for the future and a follow-up appointment or meeting can be arranged.
- Finally, you should thank the person for their time and close the session appropriately: 'Its been a pleasure speaking with you', 'I hope that helps, we can discuss it further next time'.

Top tips

→ **Taking a history**

This should include the eight classic features.

- Personal details: name, age, sex, and occupation
- PC (presenting complaint)
- HPC (history of presenting complaint): onset; duration; character; associated features; risk factors; system-specific history; investigations and treatment to date
- PMHx (past medical history) and PSHx (past surgical history)
- DHx (drug history) and allergies
- FHx (family history)
- SOHx (social and occupational history): alcohol (e.g. pancreatitis); smoking (smoking-related cancers); foreign travel (e.g. diarrhoea); asbestos exposure (e.g. mesothelioma)
- SR (systems review): cardiovascular; respiratory; gastrointestinal; urological; neurological; musculoskeletal; endocrine.

→ ## Bad news

A useful mnemonic for breaking bad news is **SPIKES**:

- **S** = **s**et stage and **s**etting
- **P** = **p**atient perception – 'ICE'
- **I** = **i**nvitation – are they prepared to discuss?
- **K** = **k**nowledge – convey bad news in small, digestible pieces and check understanding
- **E** = **e**xplore emotions and **e**mpathise – create space for reaction and listen
- **S** = **s**trategy and **s**ummary – discuss management plan and give contact details.

→ ## Consent

A useful mnemonic when consenting a patient for a procedure is **CONSENTS**:

- **C** = **c**ondition and natural history – explain the clinical condition and prognosis
- **O** = **o**ptions and alternatives – no treatment; conservative; medical; radiological; surgical
- **N** = **n**ame of procedure – official title and practically what it entails
- **S** = **s**ide-effects/complications – anaesthetic; infection; bleeding; recurrence; others (e.g. stoma formation)
- **E** = **e**xtra procedures – drain; nasogastric tube; catheter; patient-controlled analgesia; stoma formation; blood transfusion
- **N** = **n**amed person operating, plus assistants
- **T** = **t**rial and **t**raining – if part of a research trial or presence of any students
- **S** = **s**econd opinion – a second opinion may be obtained prior to consenting.

Abbreviations

AAA	abdominal aortic aneurysm	CRP	C-reactive protein
A–B–C–D–E	airway–breathing–circulation–disability–exposure	CSF	cerebrospinal fluid
		CT	computed tomography
ABG	arterial blood gas	CTPA	CT pulmonary angiogram
ABPI	ankle–brachial pressure index	CVA	cerebrovascular accident
ACE	angiotensin converting enzyme	CVP	central venous pressure
AF	atrial fibrillation	CXR	chest X-ray
AIDS	acquired immunodeficiency syndrome	DIC	disseminated intravascular coagulation
ALP	alkaline phosphatase	DIPJ	distal interphalangeal joint
ALT	alanine aminotransferase	DNA	deoxyribonucleic acid
ARDS	acute respiratory distress syndrome	DRE	digital rectal examination
AS	ankylosing spondylitis	DVT	deep vein thrombosis
ASA	American Society of Anesthesiologists	EBV	Epstein–Barr virus
ASIS	anterior superior iliac spine	ECF	extracellular fluid
AST	aspartate aminotransferase	ECG	electrocardiogram
ATLS	advanced trauma life support	ECHO	echocardiogram
AXR	abdominal X-ray	ENT	ear, nose and throat
BCC	basal cell carcinoma	ERCP	endoscopic retrograde cholangio-pancreatography
BMI	body mass index		
BP	blood pressure	ESR	erythrocyte sedimentation rate
CABG	coronary artery bypass graft	FBC	full blood count
CBD	common bile duct	FCU	flexor carpi ulnaris
CCF	congestive cardiac failure	FDP	flexor digitorum profundus
CD	Crohn's disease	FEV	forced expiratory volume
CEA	carcinoembryonic antigen	FFD	fixed flexion deformity
CMV	cytomegalovirus	FFP	fresh frozen plasma
CNS	central nervous system	FNAc	fine-needle aspiration cytology
CO	cardiac output	FPL	flexor pollicis longus
COPD	chronic obstructive pulmonary disease	FVC	forced vital capacity
		G&S	group and save
CPAP	continuous positive airway pressure	GA	general anaesthetic

GCS	Glasgow Coma Scale	NO	nitric oxide
GI	gastrointestinal	NPC	nasopharyngeal carcinoma
GTN	glyceryl trinitrate	NSAID	non-steroidal anti-inflammatory drug
HB	haemoglobin	OA	osteoarthritis
HBV	hepatitis B virus	OCP	oral contraceptive pill
HCC	hepatocellular carcinoma	OGD	oesophago-gastro-duodenoscopy
HCG	human chorionic gonadotrophin	PBC	primary biliary cirrhosis
HCV	hepatitis C virus	PCA	patient-controlled analgesia
HHV	human herpes virus	PE	pulmonary embolus
HIV	human immunodeficiency virus	PEEP	positive end-expiratory pressure
HPV	human papilloma virus	PEFR	peak expiratory flow rate
HR	heart rate	PEG	percutaneous endoscopic gastrostomy
HRT	hormone replacement therapy		
HSV	herpes simplex virus	PEP	post-exposure prophylaxis
HTLV	human T-cell leukaemia virus	PIPJ	proximal interphalangeal joint
IBD	inflammatory bowel disease	PNS	peripheral nervous system
ICD	implantable cardiac defibrillator	PR	per rectum
ICP	intracranial pressure	PSA	prostate-specific antigen
ICU	intensive care unit	PVD	peripheral vascular disease
IHD	ischaemic heart disease	RIF	right iliac fossa
IM	intramuscular	RR	respiratory rate
IPJ	interphalangeal joint	RUQ	right upper quadrant
ITP	idiopathic thrombocytopenic purpura	SCC	squamous cell carcinoma
IV	intravenous	SFJ	sapheno-femoral junction
JPS	joint position sense	SIJ	sacro-iliac joint
JVP	jugular venous pressure	SIRS	systemic inflammatory response syndrome
LDH	lactate dehydrogenase		
LFT	liver function test	SLE	systemic lupus erythematosus
LIF	left iliac fossa	SVC	superior vena cava
LMN	lower motor neuron	TB	tuberculosis
LMW	low molecular weight	TED	thromboembolic deterrent
LUQ	left upper quadrant	TGF	transforming growth factor
MCP	metacarpophalangeal joint	TIBC	total iron binding capacity
MDT	multidisciplinary team	TNF	tumour necrosis factor
MEN	multiple endocrine neoplasia	TPR	total peripheral resistance
MI	myocardial infarction	TRAM	transverse rectus abdominis flap
MRC	Medical Research Council	TSH	thyroid stimulating hormone
MRCS	Member of the Royal College of Surgeons	U&Es	urea and electrolytes
		UC	ulcerative colitis
MRI	magnetic resonance imaging	UMN	upper motor neuron
MRSA	methicillin-resistant *Staphylococcus aureus*	USS	ultrasound scan
		UTI	urinary tract infection
NG	nasogastric	VATS	video-assisted thoracoscopic surgery
NICE	National Institute for Clinical Excellence	WCC	white cell count
		WHO	World Health Organization

Index

Numbers in italics refer to Figures; those in bold type refer to Tables.